Essential Medical Procedures

Essential Medical Procedures

EDITED BY

Peter J Toghill
MD, FRCP(LOND & ED)

Director of Continuing Medical Education,
Royal College of Physicians of London, UK
and
Emeritus Consultant Physician,
Queen's Medical Centre, Nottingham, UK

A member of the Hodder Headline Group
LONDON • SYDNEY • AUCKLAND
Copublished in the USA by Oxford University Press, Inc., New York

First published in Great Britain in 1997 by
Arnold, a member of the Hodder Headline group,
338 Euston Road, London NW1 3BH

Co-published in the United States of America by
Oxford University Press, Inc.,
198 Madison Avenue, New York, NY10016
Oxford is a registered trademark of Oxford University Press

Whilst the advice and information in this book is believed to be true and
accurate at the date of going to press, neither the author[s] nor the publisher
can accept any legal responsibility or liability for any errors or omissions
that may be made. In particular (but without limiting the generality of the
preceding disclaimer) every effort has been made to check drug dosages;
however, it is still possible that errors have been missed. Furthermore,
dosage schedules are constantly being revised and new side-effects
recognized. For these reasons the reader is strongly urged to consult the
drug companies' printed instructions before administering any of the drugs
recommended in this book.

British Library Cataloguing in Publication Data
A catalogue record for this book is available from the British Library

Library of Congress Cataloging-in-Publication Data
A catalog record for this book is available from the Library of Congress

ISBN 0 340 63187 2

Composition by Scribe Design, Gillingham, Kent, UK
Printed and bound in Hong Kong by Dan Hua Printing Press Company

Contents

List of contributors

R ANDREWS MRCP(UK)
Lecturer in Cardiovascular Medicine, Queen's Medical Centre, Nottingham

A BEDLOW MRCP(UK)
Registrar in Dermatology, St George's Hospital, London

N BIENZ MRCP(UK)
Senior Registrar in Haematology, Nottingham City Hospital, Nottingham

R M CHARNLEY DM FRCS
Consultant Surgeon, Freeman Hospital, Newcastle upon Tyne

J M DAVIES MD FRCP FRCPath
Consultant Haematologist, Queen's Medical Centre, Nottingham

M DOHERTY MD FRCP
Professor of Rheumatology, Rheumatology Unit, Nottingham City Hospital, Nottingham

F FAWTHROP PhD MRCP(UK)
Senior Registrar, Rheumatology Unit, Nottingham City Hospital, Nottingham

I W FELLOWS DM FRCP
Consultant Physician and Gastroenterologist, Norfolk and Norwich Healthcare Trust, Norwich

G M FILSHIE DM FRCOG
Reader/Consultant in Obstetrics and Gynaecology, Queen's Medical Centre, Nottingham

P FORSYTH MRCP(UK)
Registrar in Haematology, Queen's Medical Centre, Nottingham

N M GAJRAJ FRCA
Senior Registrar, Department of Anaesthesia, Queen's Medical Centre, Nottingham

K P GIBBIN FRCS
Consultant, Department of Otorhinolaryngology, Head and Neck Surgery, Queen's Medical Centre, Nottingham

K J GIRLING FRCA
Lecturer in Anaesthesia, Queen's Medical Centre, Nottingham

H GOULDING MRCPath
Consultant Histopathologist, States of Jersey Pathology Laboratory, Jersey

D GRAY DM MRCP(UK)
Reader in Medicine and Honorary Consultant Physician, Queen's Medical Centre, Nottingham

I P HALL DM FRCP(UK)
Senior Lecturer in Therapeutics, Queen's Medical Centre, Nottingham

C HARLAND MRCP(UK)
Consultant Dermatologist, St Helier Hospital, Carshalton

D P HAY MB ChB
Research Fellow, Department of Obstetrics and Gynaecology, Queen's Medical Centre, Nottingham

S S HEHAR FRCS
Senior House Officer, Department of Otorhinolaryngology, Head and Neck Surgery, Queen's Medical Centre, Nottingham

G J HOBBS FRCA
Senior Lecturer in Anaesthesia, Queen's Medical Centre, Nottingham

A R HOUGHTON MRCP(UK)
Cardiology Research Fellow and Honorary Medical Registrar, Queen's Medical Centre, Nottingham

J W IACOVOU DM FRCS(Ed)
Consultant Urologist, Princess Margaret Hospital, Swindon

J LUND FRCS
Research Fellow, Department of Surgery, Queen's Medical Centre, Nottingham

H MAY MB MRCP(UK)
Senior Registrar, West Norwich Hospital, Norwich

A F MULLER DM MRCP(UK)
Consultant Physician and Gastroenterologist, Kent and Canterbury Hospital NHS Trust, Canterbury

R J POWELL DM FRCP
Consultant Clinical Immunologist, Senior Lecturer in Immunology, Queen's Medical Centre, Nottingham

N H RUSSELL MD FRCP FRCPath
Reader in Haematology, Nottingham City Hospital,
Nottingham

C D SELBY DM MRCP
Consultant in Respiratory and Intensive Care
Medicine, Queen Margaret Hospital, Dunfermline

H TERRY MRCP(UK)
Senior Registrar, Health Care of the Elderly,
Queen's Medical Centre, Nottingham

A THOMAS MRCP(UK)
Registrar in Medicine, Queen's Medical Centre,
Nottingham

P J TOGHILL MD FRCP(Lond and Ed)
Director of Continuing Medical Education, Royal
College of Physicians of London and Emeritus
Consultant Physician, Queen's Medical Centre,
Nottingham

T D WARDLE DM MRCP(UK)
Consultant Physician and Gastroenterologist,
Countess of Chester Health Park, Chester

Preface

Doctors in training are now expected to undertake an extensive variety of practical medical procedures. These vary from basic obligatory skills, such as cardiopulmonary resuscitation, to more sophisticated techniques, such as temporary cardiac pacing. The places for learning these skills are coronary care units, side wards or at the bedside, with expert tuition immediately available. There is no adequate substitute for practical experience.

Having said this, my reasons for producing this book are threefold. First, it is intended to supplement practical instruction by discussing indications, after-care and complications. Second, by adopting a detailed 'step-by-step' approach, it aims to make many of the procedures described safer and less painful for the patient. Third, it will provide the doctor working in isolation under emergency conditions with sufficient information to perform competently.

The idea for such a book resulted from a series of articles which appeared initially as a supplement to *Hospital Update*. Our SHOs and housemen found them useful and suggested that the original articles might be revised and extended to include other procedures performed by doctors during their basic medical training. I have not attempted to produce a comprehensive list but the 25 selected chapters have emerged after considerable discussion. Some procedures, such as renal biopsy or pericardial aspiration, which are normally performed in specialized units, have been deliberately excluded. It has proved virtually impossible to set out the chapters in any logical order but I have attempted to group related procedures together. Most of the chapters have been written by colleagues who work, or have worked, in Nottingham. As editor, I have attempted to blend the caution and experience of the older contributors with the technical skill and enthusiasm of the younger ones! There may be other equally safe and effective ways of undertaking these procedures, but those detailed here have been used satisfactorily in our own busy hospitals.

When I was a houseman, learning practical medical procedures, we were told, 'See one, do one, teach one!' This was very dangerous advice. Fortunately, there are now many more opportunities for young doctors to watch and learn new skills under expert supervision. We hope that this new book will be an additional stand-by.

Peter Toghill
Nottingham, 1996

Acknowledgements

It is a pleasure to acknowledge the help of many colleagues who have given their time and expertise to contribute to this book. Many of the illustrations have been prepared by the Audio-Visual Department of the Queen's Medical Centre, Nottingham and I am grateful for their help. Mrs Anne Booton of the Haematology Department of the Queen's Medical Centre gave valuable advice in Chapter 1, and Becton Dickinson have allowed us to illustrate their Vacutainer system. The algorithm on 'The Management of Pneumothorax' is reproduced by permission of the *British Medical Journal*. Guidelines for basic life support are published by permission of *Resuscitation*. Sister Lesley Reilly of the Queen's Medical Centre, Nottingham, gave considerable help in the preparation of Chapter 19.

I am particularly grateful to all the staff at Arnold who have enthusiastically undertaken this major project, and been a pleasure to work with. I am also pleased to acknowledge the help of Mrs Anne Patterson who, in her capacity as the then-Editor of *Hospital Update*, encouraged me to produce the original series of Practical Procedures as a supplement to that journal. We are indebted to the publishers of *Hospital Update* for permission to reproduce those articles, some of which have been revised and modified.

1

Venepuncture

INTRODUCTION

Venepuncture is the term used to describe puncture of a vein to obtain blood for diagnostic and analytical purposes. For most patients, this simple procedure should be virtually painless. However, if performed roughly and clumsily by an inexperienced operator, venepuncture may become a harrowing and traumatic experience. A few moments of thought and consideration at the onset may prevent unnecessary problems later on.

PRELIMINARY CONSIDERATIONS

Before a venepuncture is attempted, the following steps should be taken:

- everything needed is placed at hand;
- the patient is made warm and comfortable;
- the patient is reassured and the procedure is explained;
- a suitable vein is defined;
- a check is made about any bleeding tendency.

Site of venepuncture

In the adult, the best veins are located in the antecubital fossa (Fig. 1.1). To distend these veins, a tourniquet is placed around the upper arm. A simple elastic Velcro band is much easier to apply and release than the complex adjustable contraptions sold by some manufacturers. Tourniquet compression is limited if the patient has a haemorrhagic tendency. If the first arm examined doesn't look too hopeful, the other should be tried. If veins are difficult to find, the patient should be asked to open and close their fist

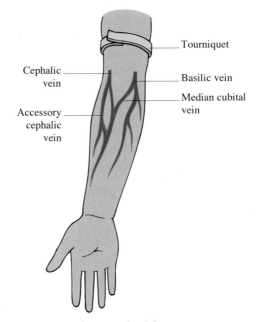

FIG 1.1   Veins in the antecubital fossa.

several times and to lower the arm so that the hand is hanging down. If necessary, the arm should be warmed by immersing it in warm water or wrapping it in a hot towel.

If possible, the vein selected is one which has not been used previously and one which is easily detected by inspection and/or palpation. A good vein should feel bouncy and will refill immediately after being compressed. Careful preliminary palpation will prevent the possibility of taking blood from an artery (which will pulsate) or of damaging a tendon. It must be remembered that the brachial artery and the median nerve are in close proximity in the antecubital fossa.

When it is not possible to find veins elsewhere, femoral venepuncture may be performed (see section below).

No attempt should be made to take blood from:

- an oedematous arm;
- possible sites of infection;
- limbs where lymphatic drainage may be impaired, such as after mastectomy;
- veins extensively damaged or thrombosed after previous venepuncture.

TECHNIQUE

Equipment

All the equipment required should be available and to hand before starting to take blood; it is more convenient to carry this to the patient in a clinically clean tray or receiver. Necessary items are:

- a tourniquet;
- a suitable syringe and needle – a 21 G needle enables blood to be withdrawn at a reasonable speed, without undue discomfort to the patient and without traumatizing blood cells;
- cotton wool balls;
- adhesive plaster or hypoallergenic tape;
- specimen bottles;
- specimen request forms.

Procedure

Gloves should be worn if the patient is in a high-risk or potentially high-risk group (see section below). A tourniquet is applied to distend the previously identified vein. At this stage (and not before), the needle guard is removed. Using the non-dominant hand, gentle traction is applied to the skin with a fingertip, a few centimetres distal to the proposed puncture site, to immobilize the vein. The syringe is held in the dominant hand with the needle bevel uppermost and the barrel almost flush with the patient's skin. As the needle enters the vein a distinct 'give' can often be felt. Before withdrawing blood into the syringe, the tourniquet is released and a few seconds allowed to elapse as blood taken during or immediately after prolonged venous occlusion may give spurious biochemical results.

After blood has been taken, the cotton wool swab is placed gently over the puncture site, the needle is withdrawn and firm pressure is applied over the site for 1 min. The arm should not be flexed to compress the swab as this predisposes to haematoma formation.

The specimen containers must be filled gently. Many samples of blood are spoiled for haematological assessment or chemical analysis by being squirted too vigorously into the containers.

THE VACUTAINER SYSTEM

The basic principles of venepuncture are used in this technique but the Vacutainer system allows blood to be taken directly into evacuated specimen tubes, thus obviating risks of spillage or contamination. The apparatus and method of use of the Becton Dickinson Vacutainer system are illustrated in Figs 1.2 and 1.3. The basic equipment (Fig. 1.2) consists of:

- a plastic disposable or a reusable needle holder, onto which the needle is attached by a screw thread;
- a double-ended needle (with a self-sealing rubber sleeve covering one end) which is screwed into the needle holder (the sleeve makes it possible for container tubes to be removed from the needle holder without contaminating it with blood);
- container tubes of various types, each with a rubber diaphragm in the cap.

Winged blood collection sets with thinner-gauge needles and Luer multisample adapters are also available; these are specifically designed for difficult veins.

The steps in the procedure are illustrated in Fig. 1.3(a–g). The white end of the needle is unscrewed, removed and discarded. The rubber-covered end is inserted into the needle holder and screwed into place. After selection and preparation of the venepuncture site as usual, the coloured section of the needle shield is removed and venepuncture is performed in the usual way. The subsequent steps are then carried out as detailed in the diagrams. When all the samples have been taken, the last tube is removed from the holder before the needle is withdrawn from the vein.

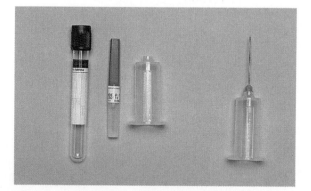

FIG 1.2 The apparatus available for the Becton Dickinson Vacutainer system of blood taking. From the left, a typical container with rubber diaphragm in the cap, the double-ended needle with the green cover protecting the bare needle and the white (or opaque) cover protecting the rubber-sleeved needle, and, the needle holder itself. On the right, the rubber-sleeved needle has been screwed into the holder and the green cover removed to expose the bare needle.

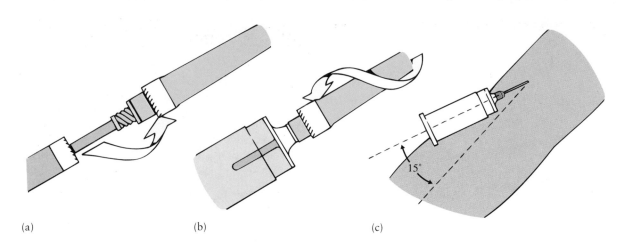

(a)   (b)   (c)

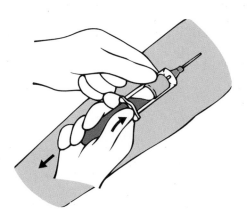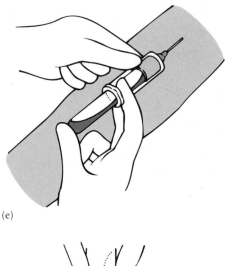

(d)   (e)

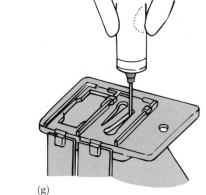

(f)   (g)

FIG 1.3   The Vacutainer system for venepuncture. (a) The paper seal is checked as proof of sterility. *If the seal is broken the needle must not be used.* Holding the coloured section of the needle shield in one hand, the white section is twisted and removed with the other hand and discarded. (b) The needle is screwed into the holder. The coloured shield is left on the needle. (c) The venepuncture site is prepared. The coloured section of the needle shield is removed. Venepuncture is performed in the usual manner with the arm in the downward position. (d) The tube is introduced into the holder. Placing the fore-finger and middle finger on the flange of the holder and the thumb on the bottom of the tube, the tube is pushed to the end of the holder, puncturing the diaphragm of the stopper. The tourniquet is removed as soon as blood begins to flow into the tube. (e) When the vacuum is exhausted and blood flow ceases, a soft pressure is applied with the thumb against the flange to disengage the stopper from the needle and to remove the tube from the holder. If more samples are needed, the procedure is repeated (from (d)). (f) While blood is flowing into succeeding tubes, the previously filled tubes containing additives are gently inverted 8 to 10 times to mix the additives with the blood. They should not be shaken. The last tube is removed from the holder before withdrawing the needle from the vein. (g) The used needle is unscrewed and discarded into the Vacutainer disposal box.

FEMORAL VEIN PUNCTURE

When it is impossible to obtain blood elsewhere, femoral vein puncture may be utilized. Here, the technique of venepuncture is different. The needle is inserted vertically to full depth into the femoral vein as it lies medial to the artery just below the inguinal ligament. If no blood appears on initial aspiration, the needle is withdrawn slowly, whilst still applying suction, until blood appears. Haemostasis is obtained by firm pressure applied to the puncture site for at least 3 min.

COMPLICATIONS

Complications of venepuncture are unusual if the procedure is performed carefully (Box 1.1). The commonest problem is local bruising, particularly in patients with bleeding tendencies.

BOX 1.1 COMPLICATIONS OF VENEPUNCTURE

Vasovagal episodes
Local bruising
Excessive bleeding from puncture site
Accidental arterial puncture
Thrombosis of traumatized vein

LABELLING SAMPLES

All sample containers must be labelled in the presence of the patient, immediately after blood has been taken. If the sample is in the 'At Risk' category, a Bio Hazard label must be attached to it and to the request form and the bag containing these (see section below).

DISPOSAL OF NEEDLES

After taking blood, needles must be discarded into an appropriately labelled and designated bin. If the Vacutainer system is used (Fig. 1.3(g)), the needle, still attached to the tube holder, is inserted into the slot of the sharps box. The needle holder is slipped to the narrow end of the slot until the needle is gripped securely. The holder is then unscrewed, allowing the needle to fall into the box. If a needle gets stuck, forceps rather than fingers should be used to unscrew and manipulate it. No attempt should be made to resheath needles. This is a dangerous procedure and is responsible for half the needlestick injuries that occur.

In the event of a needlestick injury or contamination of a cut or abrasion with blood, the following procedure should be carried out:

■ bleeding is encouraged and the injury is flushed with water (it must not be sucked);
■ the injury is washed well with soap and water;
■ a dressing is applied;
■ the injury is reported and help sought from the Occupational Health Department or the microbiologist on call.

High-risk samples

High-risk blood specimens are defined as:

■ specimens from known or suspected cases of hepatitis;
■ specimens from genitourinary clinics;
■ specimens from HIV+ patients, patients with AIDS and those suspected of having AIDS;
■ specimens from other high-risk groups;
■ specimens from patients with tropical diseases;
■ specimens leaking upon receipt.

2

Transfusion of Blood and Fluids

INTRODUCTION

The intravenous infusion of fluids or blood components is one of the most common procedures performed throughout a hospital, and it is mandatory for doctors to acquire a broad knowledge of the principles, indications and potential complications. This chapter describes the appropriate uses and some of the problems associated with the administration of blood products and intravenous fluid therapies.

The intravenous cannula is best sited in a forearm vein. Antecubital veins should not be used routinely, though they are often cannulated in emergencies in shocked patients, pending establishment of central venous access. Cannulation of veins on the dorsum of the hand should be avoided, if possible, as this site is painful, particularly with extravasation. The cannula insertion site should be protected by a transparent dressing so that it can be examined regularly for signs of infection, extravasation or superficial thrombosis. If these complications occur, the cannula should be removed and, if necessary, a fresh one sited elsewhere.

CRYSTALLOIDS AND COLLOIDS

Which fluid and when?

Consideration is given to whether the patient is water depleted (*dehydrated*), volume depleted (*hypovolaemic*), or both. If water depleted, crystalloid fluids are needed, and if volume depleted, crystalloids and colloids may be necessary. If volume depletion is

due to bleeding, red cells may be required. The aim of a 'blood transfusion' (more accurately termed a red cell transfusion) is to increase oxygen delivery to the tissues within a short time. The majority of patients with a low haemoglobin concentration are not best served by transfusion of red cells and, in some cases, red cell transfusion is likely to be more harmful than beneficial. The general state of the patient and the rate of fall of haemoglobin concentration should always be considered; anaemia which has developed over weeks or months is generally better treated by means other than red cell transfusion. However, if the patient is suffering acute blood loss, red cell transfusion will probably be necessary.

Crystalloid fluids

The main choice of crystalloid fluid lies between saline (0.9% – 'normal' saline) and glucose (5% dextrose). Normal saline contains about the same amount of sodium as plasma (150 mmol/L), whereas 5% dextrose is a way of giving water without sodium. The amount of glucose in 5% dextrose is very small (50 g/L), and it has no substantial calorific value (200 kcal/L).

The common indications for instituting crystalloid fluid therapy are as follows:

- *Replacement of lost fluid (e.g. lost through vomiting or diarrhoea).* It should be remembered that most body fluids contain salt (though less than 150 mmol/L) and potassium. Most fluid replacement regimes will therefore require the use of normal saline with potassium supplements in preference to dextrose.

TABLE 2.1 Colloid volume expanders

PRODUCT	CONCENTRATION (%)	INTRAVASCULAR PERSISTENCE	APPROXIMATE FREQUENCY OF SEVERE REACTIONS
Modified gelatin	3–4	50% at 4–5 h	1/13 000
Hydroxyethyl starch	6	>50% at 24 h	1/16 000
Dextran 70 (NB: may interfere with haemostasis and crossmatching)	6	50% at 24 h	1/5000
Human albumin	4.5	>50% at 5 days	1/30 000

■ *'Insensible' loss.* Moderate continuous sweating or fever above 39.5°C requires the addition of 500 mL normal saline and 500 mL 5% dextrose per 24 h period.

■ *Normal daily requirements.* In a 24 h period, about 2500 mL fluid, 100 mmol sodium and 70 mmol potassium are required.

In practice, most patients can be managed on fluid maintenance (per 24 h period) as follows:

■ 1 L 0.9% saline with 20 mmol potassium over 8 h;
■ 1 L 5% dextrose with 20 mmol potassium over 8 h;
■ 1 L 5% dextrose with 20 mmol potassium over 8 h.

Patients on IV fluids must have their serum urea and electrolytes measured regularly, and adjustments to the IV fluid regime made accordingly. Particular care must be taken for patients with cardiac, renal or hepatic failure, in which case more senior advice should be sought.

Colloid or crystalloid?

In the management of acute hypovolaemia, the choice of crystalloid or colloid fluid replacement remains a controversial subject. There is a theoretical increased risk of inducing pulmonary oedema with the use of crystalloid alone, by means of reducing plasma osmotic pressure and allowing 'leakage' of fluid into the extravascular space. This phenomenon is particularly encouraged in the context of septic shock, adult respiratory distress syndrome and anaphylaxis, in which there is increased vascular permeability. However, controlled trials demonstrate little difference in the outcomes of patients resuscitated with albumin solutions or crystalloid, provided that enough crystalloid is given. In practice, if more than a few litres of fluid are required in resuscitation, the use of colloid may be beneficial, especially in those situations where vascular permeability is likely to be increased.

Which colloidal solution?

There are several non-plasma-derived colloidal solutions available, the most commonly used being starch or gelatin based. The various properties are shown in Table 2.1. Human albumin solution has no specific benefit over other colloid solutions and is much more expensive; thus, its use is often restricted for specific indications, such as the treatment of severe burns, or diuretic-resistant oedema in hypoproteinaemic patients. Albumin should not be used as a substitute for IV nutrition as it is a poor source of essential amino acids. Similarly, it is not effective in the management of chronic protein loss.

RED CELL TRANSFUSION

Before ordering a red cell transfusion, the following points should be considered:

Is transfusion really necessary?

Nobody would dispute that red cell transfusion is required in the situation of massive acute blood loss, but many postoperative 'top-ups' are probably unnecessary and may expose the patient to avoidable risk. In adults, in general, a transfusion of less than 2 units of red cells is virtually never indicated, and is bad clinical practice.

What are the risks of red cell transfusion?

Non-infection risks

These can be summarized into early and late events. Early events include transfusion reactions, which can be mild (plasma protein or leucocyte reactions) or severe acute haemolytic reactions (e.g. ABO or rhesus mismatch). It should be remembered that the vast majority of life-threatening transfusion reactions occur due to clerical error: by failure to correctly identify the patient from whom the crossmatch sample was taken, failure to label the sample and request form correctly, or failure to check the identity of the recipient as the transfusion is commenced. Any red cell pack issued from the hospital blood bank carries a compatibility label with details of the patient for whom it is intended, and this must be checked carefully with the patient (including the wristband) immediately before transfusion commences. Other identification checks in the blood bank and at the point of collection will be dictated by local operational procedures.

Volume overload and concomitant heart failure are considerable risks in the elderly or very young patient requiring red cell transfusion, and can often be anticipated and treated promptly.

Late effects of transfusion include the induction of red cell alloantibodies which can render any further crossmatching more difficult, and, in the multiply transfused patient, long-term iron overload can lead to multiple organ failure.

Infection risks

The medical selection of blood donors in the UK is intended to exclude anyone whose blood might harm the recipient. For this reason, the National Blood Transfusion Service maintains a policy whereby volunteer unpaid donors are recruited and medically assessed at their first donation by a medical officer and at each subsequent donation by means of questionnaire (Box 2.1). However, red cell products are capable of transmitting any agent present in cells or plasma which for any reason has not been detected by routine donor screening. In the UK, all donated blood is tested for hepatitis B surface antigen, hepatitis C antibody, HIV-1 and HIV-2 antibodies and *Treponema pallidum* (syphilis) antibody (Box 2.1). It should be borne in mind that other infectious agents are not routinely screened for, including parasitic agents such as malaria or toxoplasma, or viral infections such as EBV, HTLV-1 and slow viruses. Also, screening by means of antibody testing will miss the transmissible agent if the donor blood is tested during the first few weeks of infection, before seroconversion occurs.

RED CELL PRODUCTS

The Regional Blood Transfusion laboratories in the UK coordinate the collection, processing, testing and supply of blood products to all hospital blood banks. The great majority of 'blood' transfusions required are red cell transfusions, and most donor units are processed at the Regional Transfusion Centre with this in mind. Plasma is separated from the donor unit at an early stage, to be stored as fresh frozen plasma (FFP), or processed for cryoprecipitate or specific coagulation factor concentrates. Thus, 'fresh whole blood' is rarely available at the hospital blood bank; in the situation of acute massive blood loss, where 'fresh whole blood' may be indicated, red cell components supplemented with fresh frozen plasma and platelet concentrates are just as effective.

Red cell products are usually supplied in the following forms:

Red cell concentrate (CPD-A1)

This product is red cells from a single donor with citrate, phosphate, dextrose, and adenine as anticoagulant. Most of the plasma has been removed and the haematocrit is high (55–75%). The red cells can be given along with normal saline via a Y-pattern giving set if flow is poor.

Red cell concentrate in optimal additive solution

In this product, plasma-reduced red cells from a single donor are resuspended in nutritive solution, usually SAG-M (saline, adenine, glucose and mannitol). The haematocrit is 50–70%, with reduced viscosity which improves the blood flow and the storage properties of the cells. This product is not recommended for exchange transfusion but is suitable for 'top-ups'.

Other red cell products

Leucocyte-depleted ('filtered') red cell products and washed red cells are also available for specific indications. Each unit of red cells transfused should be expected to raise the haemoglobin concentration by approximately 1 g/dL in an adult.

BOX 2.1 BLOOD DONORS – MEDICAL ASSESSMENT AND TESTS

All donors are non-remunerated, aged 18–70 years, weighing >50 kg

Questions
- General medical history at first donation
- Recent illnesses including recent minor febrile disorders
- Travel history – past or recent
- Recent tattoos or body piercing
- Sexual history
- Pregnancies

Tests
- Copper sulphate screening Hb, predonation
- *Treponema pallidum* antibody
- Hepatitis B surface antigen
- HIV-1 and HIV-2 antibody
- Hepatitis C antibody

INDICATIONS FOR RED CELL TRANSFUSION

The following indications account for the vast majority of red cell transfusions in the UK:

■ *Acute blood loss (trauma/surgery).* Both red cells and volume replacement are needed. Red cell concentrates and plasma expanders should be used, and, in massive blood loss, the need for fresh frozen plasma and platelet concentrate should be considered. The blood bank technician and medical haematologist are there to advise, so assistance should be requested if in doubt.

■ *Preoperative blood transfusion.* It is generally safer to correct anaemia with appropriate haematinics rather than transfuse the patient. On appropriate replacement therapy, the haemoglobin concentration is likely to rise by the order of 1 g/dL per week. In some situations, such as an emergency procedure or in the face of failure to respond to haematinics and a haemoglobin concentration of <8 g/dL, preoperative transfusion is appropriate. If the haemoglobin concentration is 8–10 g/dL, each case should be assessed individually before deciding to transfuse.

■ *Anaemia of chronic disease.* Some patients with malignancy or other chronic inflammatory process may require red cell transfusion if they are symptomatic of anaemia that does not respond to haematinics. Patients with symptomatic anaemia due to chronic renal failure are usually managed with oral iron and erythropoietin, but sometimes transfusion is also necessary.

■ *Bone marrow failure.* These patients will require transfusion with red cells and other blood components.

■ *Transfusion-dependent conditions.* This group includes severe thalassaemia, when regular transfusion is usually required from a young age, and some myelodysplastic syndromes, including sideroblastic anaemia. These patients, mainly as the result of repeated blood transfusions, will develop severe tissue iron overload; the concomitant use of the iron-chelating agent desferrioxamine will be necessary. Some patients with severe sickle cell disease also require regular transfusions to suppress their own HbS production.

Other possible indications include exchange transfusion for haemolytic disease of the newborn, or, rarely, for severe falciparum malaria or meningococcal septicaemia. Occasionally, patients with immune-mediated haemolysis may require transfusion, but this should not be undertaken without the advice of a haematologist.

ORDERING AND ADMINISTERING RED CELLS

There are minimum requirements concerning the ordering and administration of red cells; the following points are mandatory:

■ All samples and request forms must contain accurate identification with at least three points of reference, for example, full name, hospital number and date of birth.

■ Release/collection of red cell packs from the blood bank must include a locally agreed method of rechecking the patient details.

■ Blood must be stored only in designated fridges with continuous temperature monitoring and appropriate alarms. Once removed from a blood refrigerator, the red cell transfusion should be started within 30 min.

■ Immediately before administration of the red cell unit, the compatibility label must be checked with the patient identity, including the patient's wristband. Again, there must be a minimum of three points of reference. No discrepancies should be accepted.

■ Drugs must never be added to blood.

Each unit of red cells should be transfused through a designated blood giving set containing a 170 μm filter within a maximum of 4 h. The patient should be monitored during and after transfusion, according to local guidelines. Minimum observations are the recording of temperature, pulse and blood pressure every 30 min, with particularly close observation during the first 5–10 min of each unit.

How long does a crossmatch take?

There are essentially three tests necessary in the blood bank when a request for blood is received. First, the ABO and rhesus D group of the patient is defined ('grouping'). This takes a matter of 5–10 min in an emergency situation. If blood is required from the blood bank immediately, a maximum of 2 units of 'flying squad' uncrossmatched O Rh negative may be used, followed by group-compatible blood thereafter. If more time is available, the recipient's serum will be screened for the presence of any antibodies against red cell antigens ('screening'). This screening test takes a minimum of 20 min to perform. If antibody screening is negative, red cells can, in general, be safely transfused according to ABO and rhesus D group without a formal crossmatch. However, if the antibody screen is positive, there will be an *inevitable* delay of several hours in providing suitable red cells for transfusion whilst further steps to define the specific antibody are carried out. This often entails sending samples to the Regional Transfusion Centre. Full crossmatching of donor units against recipient serum is the final, safest compatibility test, is generally mandatory for all elective transfusions, and usually necessitates incubations of approximately 40–60 min. In an emergency situation, a full crossmatch generally takes 30–40 min from the arrival of appropriately labelled specimens at the blood bank.

Transfusion reactions

Recommended immediate actions in a suspected transfusion reaction are shown in Box 2.2. Acute haemolytic reactions are very rare but are life threatening. The most severe occur due to ABO mismatch, most often due to misidentification of the crossmatch sample, the recipient or the blood pack in use. Identification checks throughout the process of ordering, crossmatching, collecting and administering blood should, if carried out correctly, prevent such mishap. An acute haemolytic reaction is manifested by chest or loin pain, dyspnoea, hypotension and tachycardia, which can progress rapidly to DIC and acute renal failure. If an acute haemolytic reaction is suspected, the transfusion should be stopped immediately, the unit rechecked against the patient, copious clear fluids given and renal output monitored. The blood unit is returned to the blood bank with a further crossmatch and EDTA sample from the patient, and the blood bank staff are informed immediately.

Much more common are simple febrile or allergic reactions, due to non-specific plasma protein or leucocyte antibodies. In a simple febrile reaction, aspirin or paracetamol are given and the transfusion is slowed, but close observation of the patient continues and the transfusion is stopped if symptoms and signs do not resolve. Similarly, if an allergic reaction occurs (pruritus and/or urticaria) antihistamines should be given and further transfusion discussed with blood bank staff. If recurrent reactions occur, high-grade leucocyte filtering of the red cells may be required.

BOX 2.2   TRANSFUSION REACTIONS

Suspected acute haemolytic transfusion reactions (chest/loin pain, dyspnoea, shock). Immediate actions:

- Stop transfusion
- Keep cannula open with saline
- Check identity of patient against unit
- Send blood unit and giving set to blood bank with a fresh 20 mL clotted and 5 mL EDTA sample from the patient
- Discuss with blood bank

Febrile reactions:

- Give aspirin or paracetamol
- Observe closely until symptoms resolve
- Recommence transfusion if tolerated
- Consider leucocyte filtration of blood after discussion with blood bank

Allergic reactions (pruritus/urticaria):

- Give antihistamines/steroids as needed
- Discuss further transfusion with blood bank

USES OF OTHER BLOOD PRODUCTS

The following blood products are also available via the hospital blood bank, but usually require discussion and/or advice from a haematologist before use.

Platelet concentrate

Platelet transfusions are indicated in a patient bleeding due to thrombocytopenia or platelet function defect, and in massive transfusion. Prophylactic platelet transfusions are necessary in bone marrow failure, the threshold for transfusion usually being a platelet count less than 10×10^9/L, or less than 20×10^9/L if the patient is febrile. The usual adult dose is 5 units (1 unit is defined as containing 55×10^9/L) infused through a standard blood giving set over 30 min. The platelets should ideally be ABO compatible with the recipient but do not need to be crossmatched. A dose of 5 units of platelets should be expected to raise the platelet count by $20–40 \times 10^9$/L in an adult, providing there is no increased consumption. Platelet concentrates are stored with agitation at 20–24°C, and the shelf-life is only 5 days. Thus, large stocks are not kept in the hospital blood bank, and notice is required to request supplies from the Regional Transfusion Centre.

Fresh frozen plasma

This contains many different coagulation factors (Box 2.3) and is indicated for the replacement of multiple clotting factor deficiencies in patients with liver disease, DIC, or to correct warfarin overdosage. It is also necessary in massive transfusion as red cell products contain limited clotting factors. An initial dose of 4–6 units is appropriate in an adult, and

BOX 2.3   COAGULATION FACTORS PRESENT IN FFP

- Factor I (fibrinogen)
- Factor II (prothrombin)
- Factor V
- Factor VII
- Factor VIII (antihaemophilic factor)
- Factor IX (Christmas factor)
- Factor X
- Factor XI
- Factor XII (Hageman factor)
- Factor XIII (fibrin stabilizing factor)
- Antithrombin III
- Protein C
- Protein S
- Fibronectin

should be ABO compatible with the recipient. The FFP should be infused via a standard blood giving set as soon as possible after thawing. Moderate reactions are common, often requiring the use of antihistamines.

Cryoprecipitate

This is given to replace fibrinogen in patients with DIC or bleeding due to dysfibrinogenaemia. It is also used as an alternative to Factor VIII or XIII concentrate in the treatment of inherited deficiencies of those factors, or in von Willebrand's disease, although the specific coagulation factor concentrate should be given in preference if available. The usual adult dose is 10 units (the ABO group does not matter), and it should be infused as soon as possible after thawing.

Specific clotting factor concentrates

Freeze-dried, heat-treated concentrates of Factor VIII, Factor IX and some other coagulation factors are available for treatment of patients with inherited deficiencies of these factors. Stocks are usually kept only in designated haemophilia centres and the use of these products must always be discussed with a haematologist.

FURTHER READING

Contreras, M. (ed.) 1992: *ABC of transfusion*. London: British Medical Journal Books.

Langford, R.A., Mythen, M.C., Mann, C.V., Russell, R.C.G. and Williams, N.S. (eds) 1995: Acute resuscitation and support. In *Bailey & Love's short practice of surgery*, 22nd edn. London: Chapman and Hall Medical, 28–42.

McLelland, D.B. (ed.) 1989: *Handbook of transfusion medicine*. London: HMSO.

3

Insertion of a Central Venous Line

INTRODUCTION

Insertion of a central venous line is an invaluable aid in the management of a range of medical and surgical conditions in which problems of fluid balance or venous access occur. It is a procedure that, until mastered, tends to be underutilized, partly through fear of complications. Hence, it is important to gain experience of central venous cannulation at an early stage in training.

In addition to its value in haemodynamic monitoring, the technique of central venous cannulation is required for other practical procedures, including insertion of temporary pacing wires, Swan–Ganz catheters (to monitor pulmonary wedge pressures) and haemodialysis catheters.

INDICATIONS

Central venous cannulation should be considered in any patient who requires careful monitoring of their fluid balance. It is particularly valuable in the management of gastrointestinal haemorrhage, where a fall in central venous pressure may precede overt evidence of rebleeding. In addition, in patients with difficult venous access, central venous cannulation provides a reliable route for the administration of fluids and drugs. However, in situations where prolonged venous access is required, for example in patients who are at risk of infection, then it may be better to use a tunnelled line (i.e. one where the point of insertion into the skin is distant from the point of

BOX 3.1   SOME INDICATIONS FOR CENTRAL VENOUS LINE INSERTION

Monitoring haemorrhage
   Gastrointestinal haemorrhage and variceal bleeding
   Major trauma

Monitoring fluid balance
   Acute renal failure
   Hypovolaemia caused by severe vomiting/ diarrhoea
   Severe self-poisoning
   Acute pancreatitis
   Hyperosmolar coma and severe diabetic keto- acidosis
   Dilutional hyponatraemia (SIADH[a])

Haemodynamic monitoring[b]
   Adult respiratory distress syndrome
   Heart failure
   Septic shock

Administration of drugs[c]
   Chemotherapy (e.g. for lymphoma)
   Subacute bacterial endocarditis
   Cystic fibrosis
   Patients requiring parenteral nutrition

[a]SIADH, syndrome of inappropriate antidiuretic hormone secretion.
[b]Ideally in conjunction with monitoring pulmonary capillary wedge pressure via a Swan–Ganz catheter.
[c]Ideally through a tunnelled line (*see* Fig. 3.1).

access to the subclavian vein) to reduce the risk of infection. Some common reasons for central venous line insertion are given in Box 3.1.

ROUTES OF ACCESS

There are three common routes of access for central venous cannulation, namely the subclavian, the internal jugular and the antecubital approaches. Of these routes, the antecubital approach is unreliable because of the difficulty in feeding a long line into the intrathoracic central veins. Although there is some evidence that the risk of complications is lower with the internal jugular approach, this method is more frightening to the patient. It is, however, the route of choice for the anaesthetized patient. The subclavian approach is the most frequently used route for central venous access in the management of acute medical problems and is the method described in this chapter (Fig. 3.1).

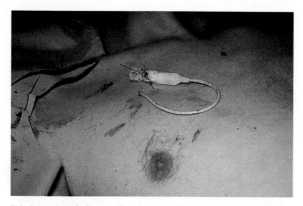

FIG 3.1 A subclavian line *in situ* for parenteral nutrition. The original point of insertion has been closed and the line tunnelled subcutaneously to emerge from the skin at a point 5 cm distant.

PRECAUTIONS AND CONTRAINDICATIONS

Often, the requirement for venous access/haemodynamic monitoring in the critically ill patient will override other considerations. The most frequent complications of the procedure are haemorrhage, pneumothorax and infection. Hence, individuals at increased risk of these complications should be evaluated carefully before cannulation is attempted. As a guide, absolute contraindications include contralateral pneumothorax, ipsilateral chest wall infection, ipsilateral arterial aneurism and ipsilateral single lung transplant. Relative contraindications include bilateral lung disease, haemorrhagic tendency

and anticoagulant therapy. The commonest worry concerns patients who are anticoagulated. One solution is to attempt to insert a long line via the antecubital route using a Drum catheter or a cut down so that direct pressure can be applied to the site of insertion to prevent bleeding. If this proves impracticable, then insertion of a subclavian or an internal jugular line may be necessary. In practice, the risk of serious haemorrhage, although increased, is still small. In patients who are overanticoagulated by heparin or warfarin, reversal of the effects of these agents can be achieved before cannulation by giving protamine or fresh frozen plasma, respectively. Vitamin K should not be given to patients requiring long-term anticoagulation as regaining control will be very difficult.

EQUIPMENT FOR AND PRINCIPLES OF CENTRAL VENOUS CANNULATION

A range of catheters is available but all use a similar design based on the Seldinger technique. The principle behind this technique is initially to gain access to the subclavian vein using a needle (the introducer), usually attached to a syringe, which may be filled with sterile saline to make it easier to mark the entry into the vein. The syringe is then removed, and a guidewire is passed down the introducer into the vein. The introducer is removed over the guidewire, leaving the guidewire *in situ* in the subclavian vein. A plastic dilator (essentially, a blunt-ended piece of hollow tubing) is sometimes used to create a track through the subcutaneous tissues, although this is necessary only for the insertion of certain types of large-bore lines. The central line itself is passed over the guidewire which is then removed, leaving only the cannula in the vein. This is then sutured to the skin and a dressing is applied. The open end of the cannula can be attached to a standard giving set for the administration of fluids, or to a manometer attached for monitoring central venous pressure.

Specialized catheters

Some specialized catheters have two or three separate lumens which can be useful if central venous pressure needs to be monitored simultaneously with pulmonary wedge pressure, or if a temporary pacing wire is also required. The Swan–Ganz catheter or pacing wire can then be inserted down separate lumina without interfering with venous access or monitoring. These catheters are more expensive than central venous lines and should be reserved for patients requiring more intensive monitoring.

TECHNIQUE OF CENTRAL VENOUS MONITORING

Preliminaries

Adequate space is needed and a bed that can be tilted is essential. A nurse with previous experience of the procedure should be present to assist. The ideal environment is a specialized room on a coronary care or high-dependency unit, or the treatment room on the ward. Premedication or prophylactic antibiotics are not usually required. The items required for the procedure are listed in Box 3.2.

BOX 3.2 ITEMS REQUIRED FOR INSERTION OF A CENTRAL VENOUS CANNULA

- Central venous pressure catheter
- Manometer and stand with attached spirit level
- Small dressing pack
- Suture (e.g. 3/0 silk)
- Sterile needle holder and scissors
- Antiseptic wash (e.g. Betadine)
- Sterile towels (×4)
- Gown, mask and gloves
- Surgical blade
- 10 mL 1% lignocaine
- 20 mL sterile N-saline
- 25 G (orange-hubbed) needle
- 21 G (green-hubbed) needle or 23 G (blue-hubbed) needle
- 10 mL syringe

Preparation of the patient

The patient should lie supine on the bed without supporting pillows. With patients who are hypovolaemic, tilting the head of the bed about 15° will help fill the central veins and aid cannulation. Some patients with heart failure will be unable to tolerate lying flat for long periods of time, and hence should be placed in the supine position at the last possible moment. The ideal point of entry into the subclavian vein is where it passes under the clavicle. In order to ease cannulation, this area should be as accessible as possible. This can be achieved by asking the patient to turn the head away from the side to be cannulated and to hyperextend the neck while keeping it rotated. A towel can be placed between the wings of the scapulae to aid positioning.

The procedure is performed in a fully sterile manner with gown and gloves being worn. An area of the chest wall large enough for the whole of the clavicle and sternal notch to be palpated (to aid localization) should be swabbed and draped.

Local anaesthesia

Before attempting to cannulate the subclavian vein, the skin should be anaesthetized with about 2 mL of 1% lignocaine using an orange-hubbed 25 G needle. In most patients, the vein is entered at a point deep to the middle third of the clavicle. Hence, the initial superficial area of anaesthesia should be about 2 cm lateral and 2 cm inferior to this position. The track down to the clavicle is then anaesthetized using about 8 mL of lignocaine through a green-hubbed 21 G needle or a blue-hubbed 23 G needle (Fig. 3.2(a)). The greatest discomfort is usually noticed in patients having inadequate anaesthesia around the clavicle so operators need to ensure that they infiltrate this area well, making sure that they aspirate before injection to ensure that the subclavian vein has not been entered.

The guidewire

While waiting for the local anaesthetic to take effect, the guidewire is checked. This has a 'stiff' and a 'floppy' end, the latter for insertion down the introducer.

Cannulation

After local anaesthesia has been achieved (about 2 min), the syringe with the attached introducer should be used to draw up 5 mL of sterile N-saline (normal saline). The skin is then nicked with a surgical blade to produce an incision wide enough to take the cannula (this eases insertion of the plastic cannula over the guidewire). The introducer with the attached syringe should then be inserted (Fig. 3.2(b)), guiding it firmly but with care, in line with the ribs towards the deep part of the clavicle, aiming for the sternal notch. By keeping gentle but continuous suction on the syringe, it is easy to recognize when the vein is entered by the flush of blood into the syringe (Fig. 3.2(c)). A faint 'give' is sometimes felt upon puncturing the vein. To enter the vein, the needle is advanced just under the clavicle, still in the same direction, trying to prevent the tip going too deep; it should be possible to proceed at a constant depth once the clavicle is reached. If the clavicle obstructs the passage of the introducer, then the tip can be 'walked down' until the bony resistance ceases and the introducer can once again be advanced. The vein should be entered deep to the clavicle. The introducer should not be advanced too far at this stage; if the vein is not entered, the introducer should be withdrawn and a parallel course followed, aiming to strike the clavicle at about 0.5 cm

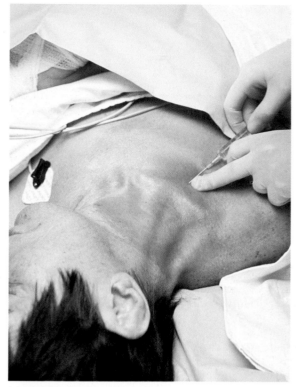

(a)

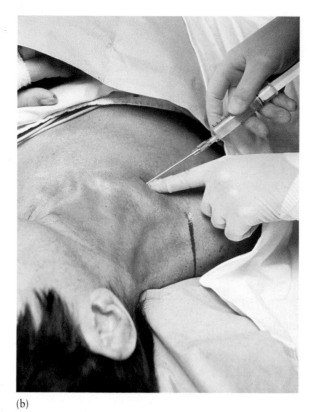

(b)

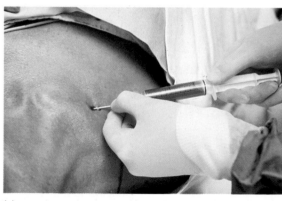

(c)

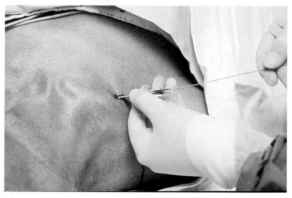

(d)

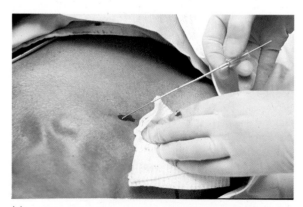

(e)

(f)

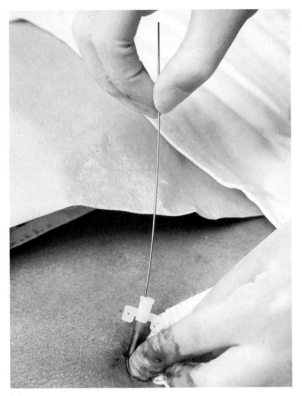

(g)

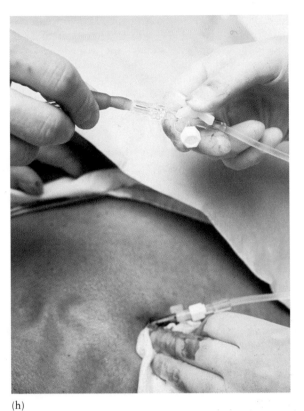

(h)

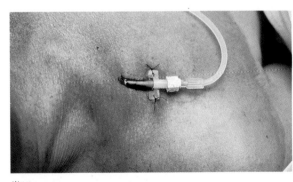

(i)

FIG 3.2   Insertion of a central venous line.

(a) The skin and subcutaneous tissues are infiltrated with local anaesthetic.
(b) The introducer, attached to the syringe, is inserted.
(c) The introducer is advanced until the vein is entered and a flashback of venous blood is obtained.
(d) The syringe is removed and the guidewire is inserted down the introducer.
(e) The introducer is removed over the guidewire.
(f) The cannula is inserted over the guidewire until flush with the skin.
(g) Guidewire is then removed leaving the cannula *in situ*.
(h) After flushing the connecting line with sterile saline, the line is attached to the cannula.
(i) The cannula is sutured to the skin.
(j) A manometer can be attached after calibrating the system to the level of the right atrium using a spirit level.

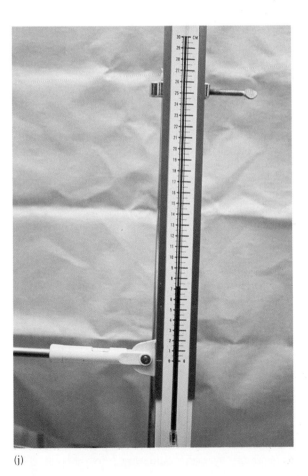

(j)

to one side of the initial attempt. This procedure is then continued until the vein is entered. If the vein cannot be found, one should not despair! In some patients, the vein may be kinked and thus be very difficult to cannulate. In these circumstances, the procedure should be handed over to a more experienced operator.

Inserting the guidewire

Once the vein has been entered, the guidewire needs to be inserted down the introducer, floppy end first. This requires some dexterity as the wire tends to uncurl (hence, the requirement of a wide sterile area) and, in addition, the syringe has to be removed from the introducer. This is best performed by holding the introducer firmly with the left hand, and gently removing the syringe. As soon as the syringe is removed, blood will flow back up the introducer; to prevent spillage, the ball of the thumb can be placed over the end of the introducer. The syringe should be placed back onto the sterile trolley and, using the right hand, the guidewire is threaded down the introducer and into the subclavian vein (Fig. 3.2(d)). The guidewire should pass easily down the vein; enough wire should be left for it to protrude from the cannula, and, if needed, for the dilator to pass over the wire and for the end of the wire to still protrude. Otherwise, when the cannula is advanced, the guidewire may be pushed irretrievably into the vein – a major disaster! The introducer should be removed over the guidewire, keeping the guidewire stationary with the left hand by holding it close to the point of entry through the skin (Fig. 3.2(e)).

Some guidewires have distance markers to help the operator judge how far they have been inserted. It is worth checking these markers against the length of the introducer before inserting the guidewire to ensure that the guidewire remains in the vein while the introducer is withdrawn.

Dilation

Central venous cannulae with a large bore (e.g. those used for insertion of a Swan–Ganz catheter) require a dilator to be used to aid insertion of the cannula. If required, the next step is to place the cannula over the dilator, which is then inserted over the guidewire. Many central venous cannulae and dilators have plastic end-stops, as part of the packaging, which need to be removed before use.

Inserting the cannula

The cannula is next advanced (complete with dilator, if required) over the guidewire into the vein (Fig.

3.2(f)). The guidewire is then removed, holding the cannula in position with the left hand, and preventing egress of blood with the thumb as the wire (and dilator, if used) is finally withdrawn (Fig. 3.2(g)). The cannula can be attached to a manometer or giving set and sutured into place (Figs 3.2(h) and (i)). Different cannulae require different sutures, but most have two small holes on the wings which can be sutured to the skin to prevent inadvertent removal. Finally, the skin is cleaned with a swab and a dressing is applied.

Postcannulation

A chest X-ray is necessary to check the position of the end of the cannula. If the cannula has been advanced too far, it can be withdrawn a few centimetres and resutured. The ideal position for the line is in the superior vena cava above the level of the right atrium.

Manometry

In order to measure central venous pressure, a manometer is attached to the end of the central venous pressure (CVP) line via a three-way tap (Fig. 3.2(j)). The manometer column is calibrated with a spirit level, using the sternal notch or the mid-axillary point as a reference point. The latter reference point is unreliable as patient rotation can result in marked variations in readings. With the patient supine, the sternal notch is between 3 and 5 cm above the level of the right atrium. The manometer column is filled with N-saline and the three-way tap is then turned to allow the manometer column alone to flow into the CVP line. Once equilibrated, the CVP level relative to the sternal notch (or, by deduction, the right atrium) can be calculated. The CVP reflects right atrial pressure, which, in turn, is related to the right ventricular end diastolic pressure (i.e. right ventricular preload). It should be remembered that in the hypovolaemic patient, vascular reflexes will tend to act to increase venous tone and hence may keep the CVP within the normal range. Any hypovolaemic insult will, however, result in an immediate fall in CVP. In patients with right ventricular failure caused by myocardial infarction affecting the right ventricle, or in patients with cor pulmonale, the CVP will be elevated.

COMPLICATIONS

There is a long list of complications for this procedure but, in practice, serious problems are very rare. Small pneumothoraces are seen in about 5% of patients but usually do not require aspiration.

Haemorrhage is unusual but may be severe, necessitating surgical intervention. Puncture of the subclavian artery also occurs in a few patients, but again serious haemorrhage is unusual. If the artery is entered, pressure should be applied over the surrounding area for at least 5 min, although this will be only partially effective as the artery lies deep to the clavicle. Relatively rare complications include puncture of the thoracic duct, brachial plexus injury, thrombosis in the superior vena cava or right atrium, air embolism, haemothorax, and arrhythmias.

PRACTICAL PROBLEMS

Several practical problems may be encountered during this procedure and a guide to these is given in Box 3.3.

BOX 3.3   PRACTICAL PROBLEMS ASSOCIATED WITH CENTRAL VENOUS CANNULATION

Problem	Solution
■ Unable to cannulate vein	■ Tilt bed with head down ■ Reposition patient ■ Try again using different entry point ■ If the above fail, try the other side of the patient
■ Unable to advance guidewire	■ Guidewire inadvertently withdrawn from vein: withdraw guidewire, reattach syringe and aspirate. If blood is obtained with ease, reattempt insertion of the guidewire. If blood is not obtained with ease, withdraw the needle and reinsert ■ Guidewire is in the internal jugular: withdraw and try again, angling the guidewire inferiorly ■ Guidewire is in the opposite subclavian: withdraw and try again, angling the guidewire inferiorly
■ Arterial blood obtained (syringe fills without suction)	■ Remove needle, apply pressure for 5 min, then try again or try the other side of the patient
■ Central venous pressure manometer fails to fall when connected	■ ? Line in subclavian artery: check partial pressure of oxygen (PaO_2) in arterial (or venous) blood from a sample from the line. If arterial, remove line and apply pressure. If venous, flush line
■ Line in right atrium on chest X-ray	■ Withdraw line by about 5 cm and X-ray again

4

Arterial Blood Sampling and Peripheral Arterial Cannulation

INTRODUCTION

Arterial puncture is performed chiefly for blood sampling and cannulation. These procedures are used routinely in clinical practice and are safe if performed with skill and care. Adequate training and experience are therefore essential, particularly for arterial cannulation. It is important to be familiar with the sites available for arterial puncture, and to understand the indications, technique and complications for each procedure.

Sites for arterial puncture

The radial artery is the usual site for arterial blood sampling and cannulation. In some patients, local trauma, burns or the type of operation being performed will determine clinical access and therefore the most appropriate site. The following superficial arteries provide the best access for arterial puncture:

- *Radial artery.* This is a branch of the brachial artery and can be palpated in the distal forearm along a line corresponding to the groove between the flexor carpi radialis tendon and the ulnar border of the tensed brachioradialis. It is most accessible immediately proximal to the wrist. Although the lumen is small (2–3 mm diameter), this site is usually clean and cannulae can be secured easily. Collateral circulation to the hand is provided by the ulnar artery.

- *Femoral artery.* This is a continuation of the external iliac and can be located in the femoral triangle distal to the mid-inguinal point (halfway between the anterior superior iliac spine and the pubic symphysis). The medial, lateral and posterior relations are the femoral vein, femoral nerve and femoral head, respectively. The femoral artery is large and has a high flow, making it the easiest site for arterial puncture and cannulation, particularly in the hypotensive or shocked patient, or when radial arterial puncture fails. Its use will usually give a more accurate measurement of blood pressure in extreme situations.

- *Dorsalis pedis artery.* This is a continuation of the anterior tibial and has a collateral blood supply to the foot. It can be palpated between the tendons of the extensor hallucis longus and extensor digitorum on the dorsum of the foot. As the artery is small, it can be difficult to puncture and is associated with a higher incidence of arterial thrombosis. It is absent in 14% of the population and gives pressure measurements higher than those in other arteries.

- *Brachial artery.* This is a larger artery and lies immediately beneath the deep fascia in the antecubital fossa. It can be palpated medial to the biceps tendon. It divides into the radial and ulnar arteries at the level of the radial neck, although division may occur at a more proximal location in the upper arm. The brachial artery may be used if arterial access cannot be obtained at other sites; however, the proximity to the elbow joint may make the continuing care of a cannula difficult.

■ *Axillary artery*. This is large but lies in close proximity to important neural structures. Furthermore, the axilla may be a difficult region to fix cannulae securely and to keep clean.

The ulnar and posterior tibial arteries can also be used. The above sites are also appropriate for use in children (Cote and Todres, 1993). In addition, the umbilical artery is used in the newborn (Kitterman *et al.*, 1970). Paediatric procedures will not be discussed further in this chapter.

ARTERIAL BLOOD SAMPLING

INDICATIONS

Arterial blood is sampled for subsequent blood gas analysis by an automated analyser. The information available from blood gas analysis is given in Box 4.1. This information provides an objective assessment of respiratory function and acid–base status. Arterial blood sampling is therefore indicated when this information may aid diagnosis or alter clinical management.

BOX 4.1 INFORMATION FROM ARTERIAL BLOOD GAS ANALYSIS

Measured parameters
- Hydrogen ion concentration (pH)
- Oxygen tension (PO_2)
- Carbon dioxide tension (PCO_2)

Calculated parameters
- Bicarbonate concentration
- Base excess
- Oxygen saturation

Respiratory function

Blood gas analysis is used to assess the adequacy of ventilation and oxygenation. For example, the type and severity of respiratory failure can be determined (e.g. CO_2 retention and dependency upon hypoxic drive or respiratory depression due to poisoning) and, in conjunction with clinical signs, the response to therapy evaluated.

Acid–base status

Acute respiratory and metabolic changes in the acid–base balance can be assessed by arterial blood gas analysis. This will be useful in patients with diabetic ketoacidosis, lactic acidosis from sepsis and shock, acute renal failure from any cause, and during the management of cardiopulmonary resuscitation. Tissue hypoxia may occur despite normal ventilation and oxygenation, giving rise to a metabolic acidosis. This may be caused by reduced tissue oxygen delivery (e.g. myocardial failure), or defective tissue oxygen utilization (e.g. cyanide poisoning). Blood gas analysis can be used to aid diagnosis and assess severity in these situations.

TECHNIQUE

Equipment

Arterial puncture for blood sampling is performed using an aseptic technique. Figure 4.1 shows the equipment required. The use of a small needle may produce less discomfort for the patient although the time for blood sampling will be longer. The use of a 23 G or smaller-gauge, sharp bevelled needle is recommended, although the use of a larger and longer needle is recommended for femoral arterial puncture. A heparinized syringe is required to prevent clotting of the sample, both in the syringe and in the analyser. A small volume of heparin (1000 units/mL) should be drawn up to coat the walls of the syringe, and all but that remaining in the syringe dead space discarded (about 0.1 mL). Prepacked heparinized syringes are available but are more expensive.

Preparing the patient

If appropriate, the patient should be informed of the reason, conduct and complications of arterial puncture. Patients may experience some discomfort with this procedure. An assistant should help position the patient in either the supine or semi-reclined

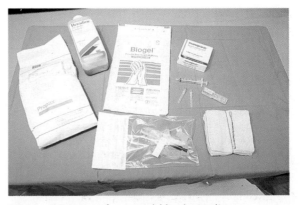

FIG 4.1 Equipment for arterial blood sampling.

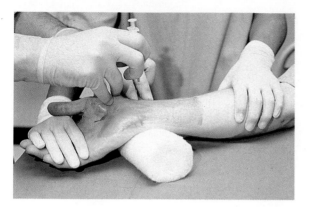

FIG 4.2 Sampling from the radial artery. Note the position of the wrist and the technique for palpating the artery.

position. Like other procedures, it is inadvisable for the patient to sit up as there is always a risk of a vasovagal response. For radial arterial puncture, the patient's wrist is gently extended and supinated by the assistant (Fig. 4.2).

Arterial puncture and blood sampling

After preparing the patient, the location of the artery is confirmed by palpation, the site is cleaned with disinfectant, and protective gloves are donned. The skin over the proposed puncture site can be injected with a small bleb of local anaesthetic; an alternative is to apply EMLA cream to the skin 1 h prior to the procedure. The use of local anaesthetic should make the procedure more comfortable, but will not prevent the pain of arterial wall puncture. The artery is then 'fixed' using the index and middle fingers of the non-dominant hand, and the needle (with heparinized syringe assembled) is introduced through the skin at an angle of 90° (Fig. 4.2). The needle is then passed through the wall of the artery while warning the patient that this may be uncomfortable. Entry into the arterial lumen will be confirmed by spontaneous filling of the syringe. In some cases, this may require gentle manual assistance, although there is a risk of obtaining a venous blood sample using this technique.

After approximately 2.0 mL of blood has been obtained, the needle should be withdrawn and firm pressure immediately applied to the puncture site, by the assistant, using a piece of gauze. The temptation to examine or 'dab' the site repeatedly should be avoided as this will increase the risk of a haematoma or bruising. Pressure should be applied for about 5 min before further examination. After this time, the site can be inspected carefully to confirm the absence of bleeding or haematoma formation. A dressing can then be applied, if necessary.

The needle should be disposed of safely, the syringe capped and labelled after air bubbles have been excluded, and the sample analysed immediately. If analysis is delayed for any reason (e.g. transport to the laboratory), the syringe should be stored in ice. This reduces the rise in $P\text{CO}_2$, and fall in $P\text{O}_2$ and pH due to continuing cell metabolism (Biswas *et al.*, 1982).

There are newer techniques available to measure continuously blood gas parameters (Hanning and Bone, 1990). Pulse oximetry is now used routinely to provide arterial oxygen saturation. Oxygen saturation can also be measured using an intravascular fibre-optic catheter. Blood gas tensions can be measured transcutaneously; these are most often performed in paediatric practice. Other developments include continuous blood gas measurement by miniature electrodes *in vivo* or mass spectrometry via a fine-bore intra-arterial cannula and tubing. Other than pulse oximetry, these techniques are expensive, can be associated with technical difficulties and are not yet used commonly in clinical practice.

Sample analysis

Most modern analysers require a 0.2 mL blood sample. As more than one sample may be required to confirm results, it is wise to obtain sufficient blood (2.0 mL) for multiple analyses. The sample should be agitated gently to ensure proper mixing immediately prior to analysis.

COMPLICATIONS

Although there are a number of potential complications of arterial blood sampling, this is a safe procedure if a sound technique is used. The most common immediate and late complications are given in Box 4.2.

Pain is common and can be minimized with experience, careful technique and the use of local

---

BOX 4.2   COMPLICATIONS OF ARTERIAL PUNCTURE

Immediate
- Pain
- Failure
- Venous sampling
- Haematoma

Late
- Ischaemia
- Infection

anaesthesia (see above). Failure is associated similarly with inexperience and poor technique. Venous sampling may occur at any site and is usually obvious. If unrecognized, it will give misleading results. Therefore, if the colour or analysis of a blood sample raises any doubt, or the oxygen saturation does not compare to a pulse oximeter reading, it is wise to repeat the procedure before taking clinical action. A haematoma may form if haemostasis is not ensured (see above). This may cause unnecessary discomfort after the procedure. Care should be exercised in the patient with a coagulopathy. In these patients, cannulation of a superficial and easily compressed arterial site, such as the radial, is good practice.

Late complications are uncommon but include distal ischaemia and infection. Ischaemia may be caused by thrombosis, embolism or spasm of the vessel. The use of the dorsalis pedis artery is not advisable in diabetic patients as there is a likelihood of poor peripheral perfusion and a risk of ulceration. The risk of infection can be reduced by using an aseptic technique, and a new needle if repeated attempts are required.

PERIPHERAL ARTERIAL CANNULATION

INDICATIONS

Invasive blood pressure monitoring dates back to 1733 when a neck artery of a horse was cannulated and connected to a vertical tube. In humans, a leg artery was first cannulated for this purpose in France in 1856. The discovery of heparin in 1917 and subsequent technical developments with plastics and electronics have facilitated the use of arterial cannulation, in particular that of the radial artery (Barr, 1961; Lambert and Wood, 1946), for invasive blood pressure monitoring. Arterial cannulation is also used increasingly for interventional radiological procedures, most frequently for vascular disease (Box 4.3).

BOX 4.3 INDICATIONS FOR ARTERIAL CANNULATION

Monitoring
☐ Frequent blood gas sampling
☐ Invasive arterial pressure monitoring

Intervention
☐ Radiological techniques
☐ Access for renal support

Monitoring

Arterial cannulation is indicated in patients who require frequent blood gas sampling and/or continuous and accurate arterial blood pressure monitoring. This is likely in the critically ill, patients undergoing deliberate hypotension, and those with unstable cardiorespiratory function or where extreme changes in blood pressure are anticipated. Therefore, arterial cannulation is a common procedure in intensive care units and operating theatres, and occasionally in coronary care units.

Intervention

Access to the arterial circulation is required for diagnostic procedures such as arteriograms, as well as therapeutic procedures such as angioplasty and embolization of intracranial aneurysms. Access is usually obtained via the larger femoral artery using a Seldinger technique (Seldinger, 1953). These procedures are obviously performed by specialist clinicians. Continuous arteriovenous haemofiltration has been used for renal support, most commonly using the femoral vessels, although this technique has been largely replaced by continuous venovenous haemofiltration.

TECHNIQUE

Equipment

In addition to the equipment shown in Fig. 4.1, appropriate cannulae and a continuous flushing and pressure monitoring system are required for peripheral arterial cannulation. There are a number of different cannulae available (Fig. 4.3). Venous cannulae are often used, but others are designed specifically for arterial use and have a guidewire to allow a Seldinger technique of insertion. The use of a guidewire may allow easier cannula insertion with less arterial wall trauma. Cannula size is important and should be adequate for performance (both blood sampling and pressure monitoring) but small enough to allow sufficient arterial blood flow whilst minimizing the risk of arterial wall damage. Furthermore, the incidence of local thrombosis increases with cannula size. For routine use in adult patients, 20 G cannulae are most frequently used. For femoral arterial cannulation, 18 G cannulae of greater length may be used. Cannulae should have parallel sides and be Teflon coated to reduce the risk of thrombogenesis.

Cannula insertion

It has been traditional practice to perform Allen's test prior to radial arterial cannulation to assess the

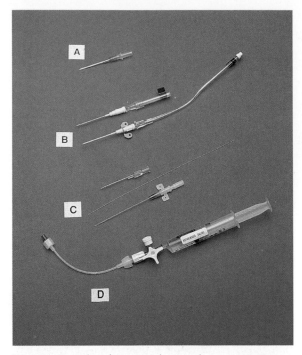

FIG 4.3 Cannulae for arterial cannulation. (A) Venous cannula. (B) Short and long Seldinger-type cannulae with integral guidewires. (C) Seldinger-type cannula with separate guidewire. (D) A 'three-way tap' and tubing primed with heparinized saline used for temporary attachment and flushing of an arterial cannula.

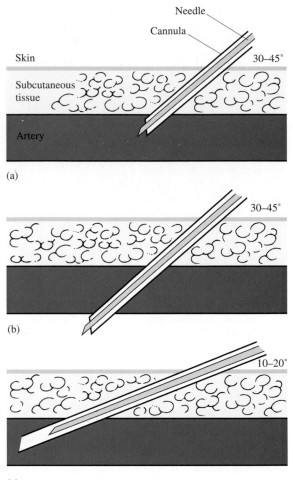

FIG 4.4 Techniques for cannulae insertion. (a) Needle placed in arterial lumen. (b) Alternative transfixion technique. (c) Cannula advanced into arterial lumen.

adequacy of collateral blood flow to the hand. It has now been established that ischaemic complications are not related to the findings of this test and its use therefore makes no real contribution to clinical practice (Wilkins, 1985). However, it is essential to observe the cannulated limb regularly for signs of ischaemia.

The procedure for arterial cannulation is conducted initially as for arterial blood sampling. Strict asepsis is essential. As the procedure can cause significant discomfort, it is sound practice in conscious patients to provide local anaesthesia, using either lignocaine injected subcutaneously over the intended puncture site or applying EMLA cream prior to the procedure. Although this will prevent the pain associated with skin and subcutaneous tissue puncture, it will not usually prevent the pain from arterial wall puncture.

The skin and artery should be punctured at an angle of about 30–45° over the site of maximum pulsation. A 'flashback' of blood indicates successful puncture. The cannula assembly is then lowered to a more acute angle and the cannula advanced over the needle into the arterial lumen. An alternative technique is to transfix the artery with the needle before withdrawing it into the lumen and passing the cannula. This is a successful alternative technique but obviously punctures the arterial wall at two sites.

Figure 4.4 demonstrates these techniques. If a guidewire is used, this is advanced through the needle into the arterial lumen and the cannula is then advanced over the wire. The wire and cannula should move freely into the arterial lumen. Difficulty threading the cannula into the artery is a common problem and may indicate needle misplacement, cannula impingement on the arterial wall, too large a cannula, or abnormal anatomy (e.g. atheroma). If blood flow from the needle is confirmed, rotation of the needle through 180° may overcome the difficulty. If not already in use, a guidewire technique should be considered. However, if there is prolonged difficulty, or if spasm of the artery or a haematoma develops, the attempt should be abandoned and immediate pressure applied to the puncture site. Further attempts can be made at another site after haemostasis. There is now a piece of equipment available that uses an ultrasonic probe to locate peripheral vessels accurately.

Connection to a continuous flushing device

After the cannula has been placed successfully, the artery is occluded proximal to the end of the cannula using firm pressure with a finger, the needle is withdrawn and the cannula is connected to the continuous flushing system (Fig. 4.5). This system delivers heparinized saline (1 unit/mL) from a pressurized bag (about 300 mmHg) at a rate of approximately 3 mL/h. This reduces the incidence of arterial thrombosis and catheter-related infection, maintains cannula patency, and prevents reflux of arterial blood. It is essential to expel all the air from the system and to use Luer-lock connections to prevent disconnection. Air in the system can cause inaccurate measurements and embolize to the circulation. The cannula should be secured with an appropriate dressing and a suture, if preferred. The dressing should ideally be clear to allow regular inspection of the cannula site.

Continuous pressure measurement

The saline-filled tubing is also part of an electronic pressure transduction system (Fig. 4.5). A hydraulic signal (transmitted from the arterial blood via the saline-filled tubing) is converted to an electrical signal by a transducer. The transducer is commonly a disposable unit incorporating a diaphragm coupled to a wire strain gauge of Wheatstone bridge configuration; the diaphragm separates the fluid column from the electrical components. Oscillations of the stiff, low-compliance diaphragm change the electrical resistance of the strain gauge and therefore the electrical signal. This signal is amplified and displayed continuously on an oscilloscope. The systolic, diastolic and mean pressures can be measured, as well as heart rate.

The pressure waveform can be distorted by inertia and friction in the fluid system from the artery to the transducer. The physical characteristics of the cannula and tubing, and the presence of air, are therefore important determinants of the accuracy of the system (Parbrook and Gray, 1990). The use of a rigid cannula with parallel sides, thick-walled tubing of limited length and internal diameter of 1.5–3.0 mm, and the meticulous exclusion of air bubbles from the system are essential to prevent signal damping. Before measuring pressures, the transducer must be placed and secured at an appropriate patient reference point and the system calibrated (*see* Fig. 4.5). If an electronic pressure transduction system is not available, the cannula can be attached via a fluid column to a simple aneroid manometer. This will provide an accurate mean pressure only.

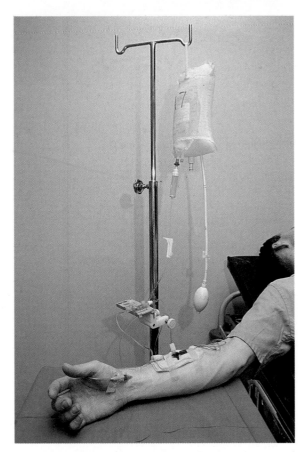

FIG 4.5 Apparatus for continuous flushing device and pressure measurement. The transducer (attached to the stand) is placed at the level of the left ventricle. The system is calibrated or 'zeroed' to atmospheric pressure by turning the three-way tap (on the forearm) off to the patient but open to the atmosphere. The transducer is then balanced electronically. When calibrated (reading is '0'), the tap can be opened to the patient and measurements started.

Taking samples from indwelling cannulae

This must be performed using an aseptic technique. A small amount of blood representing cannula 'dead space' is discarded before collecting the sample for analysis. The sample should not be withdrawn rapidly by applying a negative pressure as this can cause damage to the arterial wall and reduce the lifespan of the cannula. After sampling, the system should be flushed carefully to prevent clotting of blood in the cannula or tubing and to avoid air embolism.

COMPLICATIONS

Complications of peripheral arterial cannulation may be related to actual arterial puncture (procedural) or

BOX 4.4 COMPLICATIONS OF ARTERIAL CANNULATION

Procedural
- Pain
- Failure
- Haematoma

Cannula-related
- Haemorrhage
- Infection
- Ischaemia
- Occlusion
- Inaccurate information
- Inappropriate use

to the presence of the cannula in the artery (Box 4.4). Procedural complications are similar to those associated with arterial blood sampling; however, as the cannula is larger there is a greater risk of pain, failure and haematoma. Cannula-related complications are potentially more serious but are uncommon. Cannulae sites must be inspected regularly for signs of infection, such as inflammation or tenderness, and distal ischaemia. If there is any doubt, the cannula should be removed and resited elsewhere. Temporary blanching of local tissue may occur with flushing of the cannula and is of no clinical significance. Cannula occlusion, partial or complete, may occur from kinking or thrombosis. This will be associated with an inability to flush the cannula, failure to obtain blood samples and inaccurate or absent pressure measurements. This may be remedied by removing the faulty cannula over a new guidewire and replacing it with a new cannula, but this usually requires resiting of the cannula. As morbidity increases with the duration of use, some clinicians recommend elective resiting of cannulae at regular intervals (e.g. every 5 days). The overall incidence of complications is similar for radial and femoral arterial cannulation, although infection may be more common with the latter (Russell *et al.*, 1983).

Disconnection can be associated with significant blood loss and serious consequences, especially in children. Again, all connections must be of the Luer-lock type. Inappropriate use of the arterial cannula can be disastrous. Gangrene has been reported as a consequence of inappropriate arterial injection of an antibiotic. All arterial cannulae should be clearly labelled as such (including colour coding in red) to prevent accidental injection of substances intended for intravenous use.

The benefits of arterial blood sampling and cannulation invariably outweigh the associated risks. There are no absolute contraindications although needle entry through infected or traumatized tissue should be avoided, and arteries with a collateral circulation used preferentially.

REFERENCES

Barr, P.O. 1961: Percutaneous puncture of the radial artery with a multipurpose Teflon catheter for indwelling use. *Acta Physiologica Scandinavica* 51, 343–7.

Biswas, C.K., Ramos, J.M., Agroyannis, B. and Kerr, D.N.S. 1982: Blood gas analysis: effect of air bubbles in syringe and delay in estimation. *British Medical Journal* 284, 923–7.

Cote, C.J. and Todres, I.D. 1993: Procedures. In Cote, C.J., Ryan, J.F., Todres, I.D. and Goudsouzian, N.G. (eds) *A practice of anaesthesia for infants and children*, 2nd edn. London: W.B. Saunders, 289–304.

Hanning, C.D. and Bone, M.E. 1990: Blood gas analysis and oxygen measurement. In Scurr, C., Feldman, S. and Soni, N. (eds) *Scientific foundations of anaesthesia*, 4th edn. Oxford: Heinemann Medical Books, 119–30.

Kitterman, J.A., Phibbs, R.H. and Tooley, W.H. 1970: Catheterisation of umbilical vessels in newborn infants. *Pediatrics Clinics of North America* 17, 895.

Lambert, E.H. and Wood, E.H. 1946: Direct determination of man's blood pressure on the human centrifuge during positive acceleration. *Federation Proceedings* 5, 59.

Parbrook, G.D. and Gray, W.M. 1990: The measurement of blood pressure. In Scurr, C., Feldman, S. and Soni, N. (eds) *Scientific foundations of anaesthesia*, 4th edn. Oxford: Heinemann Medical Books, 70–81.

Russell, J.A., Joel, M., Hudson, R.J., Mangano, D.T. and Schlobohm, R.M. 1983: Prospective evaluation of radial and femoral artery catheterisation sites in critically ill adults. *Critical Care Medicine* 11, 936–9.

Seldinger, S.I. 1953: Catheter replacement of the needle in percutaneous arteriography. *Acta Radiologica* 39, 368–70.

Wilkins, R.G. 1985: Radial artery cannulation and ischaemic damage: a review. *Anaesthesia* 40, 896–9.

Temporary Cardiac Pacing

INTRODUCTION

Temporary cardiac pacing is a commonly performed procedure and is a skill eagerly sought by most junior physicians. Although temporary pacing may be life saving, it has an associated complication rate of up to 50% (Box 5.1). Many of these complications are avoidable and are a consequence of operator inexperience. Careful operative technique will usually ensure an uncomplicated procedure.

BOX 5.1   COMPLICATIONS OF VENOUS PUNCTURE AND TEMPORARY PACING

Complications of venous puncture
- Pneumothorax
- Arterial puncture
- Haemothorax
- Thoracic duct injury
- Brachial plexus injury

Complications of pacing electrode
- Thrombophlebitis
- Septicaemia
- Thromboembolism
- Myocardial perforation
- Pericarditis
- Diaphragmatic pacing
- Loss of pacing

INDICATIONS

Box 5.2 shows the more common indications for temporary pacing. In some of these situations, temporary pacing may be life saving (e.g. high-grade atrioventricular block and symptomatic bradycardia), but in many instances it will be for symptomatic (e.g. sinoatrial disease) or prophylactic (e.g. left-bundle branch block acquired during anterior infarction) reasons only. In these latter circumstances, the decision to undertake temporary pacing will be dependent upon the experience of the operator and the risks of both the arrhythmia and procedure to the patient.

BOX 5.2   INDICATIONS FOR TEMPORARY PACING

Bradycardia due to conduction tissue disease
- Symptomatic 2°/3° atrioventricular block
- Symptomatic sinoatrial disease

Acute myocardial infarction
Anterior infarction
- 3° atrioventricular block
- 2° atrioventricular block
- Alternating left/right-bundle branch block
- Right-bundle branch block, 1° atrioventricular block and left anterior/posterior hemiblock

Inferior myocardial infarction
- 2°/3° atrioventricular block with haemodynamic compromise

Ventricular tachycardia
- Ventricular overdrive/underdrive pacing in refractory cases

TECHNIQUE

Venous insertion for temporary pacing

The optimal route for temporary pacing is not certain. The British Cardiac Society recommendation is the right internal jugular vein which largely avoids the risk of pneumothorax and thoracic duct damage, and allows compression if there is inadvertent arterial puncture. It is generally the method of choice. Despite this, the right subclavian vein remains by far the preferred route within the UK. This probably reflects its ease of access, regardless of the higher risk of complications. Ultimately, the chosen route will reflect the experience of the operator and considerations of each individual patient. In kyphotic or emphysematous patients, access to the subclavian vein may be difficult or hazardous because of the risk of pneumothorax; in some elderly patients, the subclavian artery may be tortuous and anterior to the vein, restricting access. Equally, the internal jugular approach may prove difficult in 'bull-necked' individuals. Ideally, the operator should be comfortable with either approach, and that utilized should reflect each set of circumstances.

Temporary pacing after thrombolysis/anticoagulation

Accidental arterial puncture in these circumstances clearly may be especially hazardous to the patient. The route of access must be a vessel that is easily compressible and therefore the subclavian approach should be avoided. The choice lies between the femoral, median basilic, and internal and external jugular veins. The femoral vein is large, easily punctured and usually allows straightforward electrode positioning within the right ventricular apex, and is usually the preferred route. Prolonged periods of pacing (48 h) from this route are best avoided because of a risk of thromboembolism of up to 50%. The median basilic vein is a useful alternative. It is readily accessible in most patients, it is easily compressible and its localization is not hindered by an absent arterial pulse. Its use does require the patient to lie supine but it is remote if pacing is required during resuscitation. The disadvantages of this approach are occasional difficulties in electrode passage through the venous system and a slightly increased risk of electrode displacement from the right ventricular apex.

Equipment and preparation

For a successful procedure, it is essential that the correct equipment is immediately to hand and the patient is positioned appropriately. Box 5.3 shows the required equipment. Sedation is not usually required. If the subclavian or internal jugular approaches are used, then the patient should be positioned with 10–20° of head-down tilt to engorge the vein and to reduce the risk of air embolism.

The relevant area should be cleansed with iodine (or equivalent) and the patient draped with large

BOX 5.3   EQUIPMENT FOR TEMPORARY PACING

■ Large sterile towels
■ Skin-cleansing agent
■ 21 G or 18 G needle
■ 5–10 mL 1% lignocaine
■ 10 mL syringe (×2)
■ Small gallipot (×2)
■ 50 mL sterile water
■ Gauze swabs (×5)
■ No. 11 scalpel
■ 18 G Seldinger needle
■ 30–60 cm small J-guidewire
■ 5–6 French gauge haemostatic sheath
■ 5–6 French gauge bipolar temporary pacing electrode
■ Pacing box
■ Connecting leads
■ Image intensifier

surgical towels, exposing only a small operative site. After instillation of local anaesthetic, venous puncture should be performed using an 18 G Seldinger needle through which a 3 mm 'J'-curve-tipped guidewire should be passed without resistance. Fluoroscopy is then used to confirm satisfactory placement of the guidewire. If the jugular or subclavian approaches are used, then venous (rather than arterial) puncture can be confirmed by demonstration of the passage of the guidewire below the level of the diaphragm. A 5–7 French gauge haemostatic introducer sheath is then passed over the guidewire into the vein and the guidewire is removed.

The best temporary pacing electrodes are bipolar, 5–6 French gauge, with a degree of stiffness to allow easy manipulation (Fig. 5.1). Often the tip of the pacing electrode is overly acute which hinders placement in the right ventricular apex, and this is best straightened to an angle of 20° before insertion. The electrode should be advanced to the mid-right atrium (Fig. 5.2(a)). Usually, the tip will point away from the tricuspid valve towards the atrial free wall. Rotation of the electrode through 180° between thumb and forefinger will cause the tip to point towards the tricuspid valve (Fig. 5.2(b)). Advancement will then usually cause the tip to pass through the tricuspid valve, along the floor of the right ventricle into its apex (Fig. 5.2(c)). If difficulties are encountered crossing the tricuspid valve, then removal of the wire and refashioning of the bend at the tip (usually less bend) is often successful. The alternative method is by gentle advancement to create a large 180° loop within the right atrium, with the tip directed to the free wall. Rotation of the electrode through 180° between thumb and forefinger will cause the tip to 'flick' through the tricuspid valve into the right ventricle. Electrode placement within the coronary sinus is a common pitfall. It may appear to

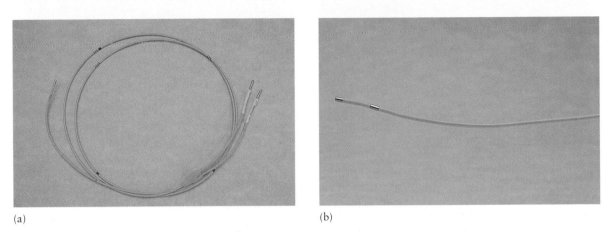

(a) (b)

FIG 5.1 A 5–6 French gauge bipolar temporary pacing electrode: (a) complete unit; (b) with tip straightened.

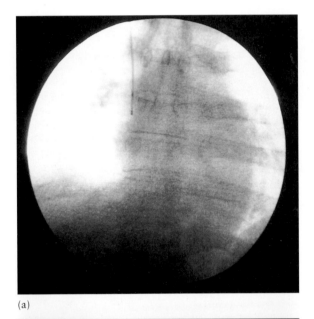

(a)

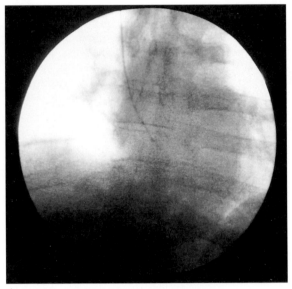

(b)

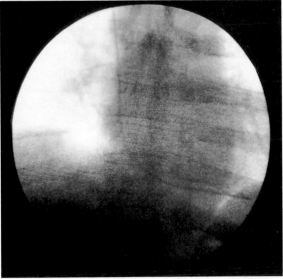

(c)

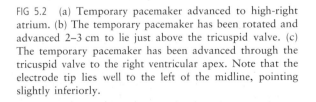

FIG 5.2 (a) Temporary pacemaker advanced to high-right atrium. (b) The temporary pacemaker has been rotated and advanced 2–3 cm to lie just above the tricuspid valve. (c) The temporary pacemaker has been advanced through the tricuspid valve to the right ventricular apex. Note that the electrode tip lies well to the left of the midline, pointing slightly inferiorly.

be within the right ventricle but the tip will be directed superiorly and posteriorly, and ventricular pacing at an acceptable voltage will not be achievable.

Pacing

Once satisfactory electrode position has been achieved, the distal pacing terminals should be securely fastened to the connecting cable and pacing box. The pacing threshold is the lowest pacing voltage that causes ventricular depolarization. This is determined by setting the pacing box at a rate 10–20% above the patient's intrinsic rate. The output is adjusted to a level sufficient to produce ventricular capture (i.e. a ventricular complex immediately after a pacing spike) and the voltage reduced slowly until ventricular capture is lost – the lowest voltage at which capture occurs is the threshold, and ideally this should be less than 1 V. The pacing box is usually left in the demand mode, with the output set at two times the threshold. A stable pacing position is ensured by observing continued ventricular capture with the patient sniffing, coughing and performing deep inspiration. The electrode is secured using 2/0 silk with one or two loops under a dressing e.g. Melolin and Mefix.

PACEMAKER FOLLOW-UP

An AP chest X-ray should be obtained immediately postprocedure to check lead position and the absence of pneumothorax. The pacing threshold should be measured and lead connections tightened daily. The insertion site must be inspected for signs of infection. Regular cardiovascular examination is, of course, essential, looking particularly for signs of pericarditis. Local infection and a rise in threshold to 4 V usually requires a new wire or repositioning. The indication for temporary pacing should be reviewed daily. In conducting tissue disease, temporary pacing is stopped when permanent pacing is instituted. Temporary pacing after myocardial infarction may be required for as long as 2 weeks before normal conduction is restored. A period of at least 24 h of pacemaker independence is required before the electrode is removed.

LOSS OF PACING

This may be life threatening and immediate action is required. Therefore, one should:

- check that the pacemaker is on;
- check all connections;
- check battery power (if applicable);
- increase output voltage to maximum (perforation or displacement will lead to an acute rise in threshold);
- switch to fixed rate (to prevent false inhibition by possible external electrical activity);
- reverse electrode polarity in case of perforation;
- attempt 'blind' repositioning if all else fails.

6

Skin Suturing

INTRODUCTION

Unless a career in surgery is pursued, most doctors will only be called upon to suture wounds of the skin following trauma or minor surgical or medical procedures. The scar is the only part of an operation that the patient will see, but, as well as providing a good cosmetic result, efficient wound closure will encourage quick healing with no wound discharge, little pain and less chance of infection.

ASSESSMENT OF A WOUND BEFORE CLOSURE

Wounds are either clean (made under sterile conditions with surgical instruments) or contaminated (made by non-sterile objects, incorporating non-sterile foreign materials or having non-viable edges after trauma). Wounds made under sterile conditions can be closed without further preparation. Contamination in dirty wounds must be eliminated before closure in order to avoid infection. If a wound is dirty, it is essential to ensure that the patient's tetanus immunization status is brought up to date.

In preparing a wound for closure:

- Haemorrhage should be controlled by applying pressure directly on the bleeding point. Haemostatic clips should never be used as there is risk of damage to other structures. The use of tourniquets is contraindicated. If bleeding does not stop after application of pressure, this may indicate that it is arising from a deeper structure and expert help should be sought.

- An assessment is made of damage to other structures, such as viscera, bone, nerves, major blood vessels or tendons. Suspected injury to any of the above requires referral to a more experienced person.
- X-rays must be taken if fragments of metals or glass might be buried in the wound.

CHOICE AND USE OF ANAESTHETIC

General anaesthesia is used for small children, patients with multiple wounds, and large or deep wounds which require extensive examination or debridement. After cleaning the wound with antiseptic solution and creating a sterile field, the wound is infiltrated with local anaesthetic. Prior to each injection, the plunger is drawn back to prevent direct intravascular injection. A 25 G or dental needle will minimize discomfort and tissue trauma. The correct plane for infiltration is in the layer of subcutaneous fat, as close to the dermis as possible. Nerves supplying the skin travel in this layer (Fig. 6.1). Lignocaine or bupivacaine are commonly used but care must be taken not to exceed the maximum dose (see Table 21.1, p. 115). Local anaesthetic incorporating adrenaline at a concentration of 1/200 000 is very effective in controlling minor oozing. The resulting vasoconstriction allows less systemic absorption of the anaesthetic and therefore higher doses may be used. Local anaesthetic containing adrenaline should *never* be used in the fingers, toes or other appendages, including ear lobes, tip of the nose or the penis, where constriction of end arteries may cause tissue ischaemia and necrosis. Time for anaesthesia to take effect should be allowed; this may be 10–15 min if

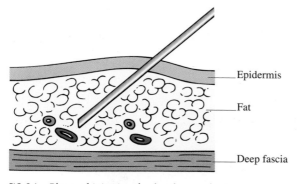

FIG 6.1   Plane of injection for local anaesthesia.

Epidermis

Fat

Deep fascia

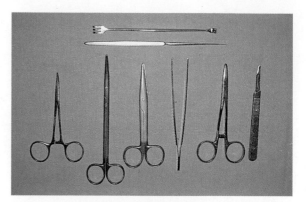

FIG 6.2   Instruments required for closure of minor wounds.

bupivacaine is used. Before going on to the suturing, absence of skin sensation should be confirmed by using the tip of a needle.

PREPARATION OF THE WOUND

After local anaesthesia, the wound can be inspected more thoroughly and, if necessary, foreign bodies removed. If important structures are seen in the wound they should be examined carefully for damage which may not have been apparent upon earlier examination (e.g. partial rupture of a tendon). Deep wounds should be washed thoroughly with copious saline and cleaned with antiseptic solution. A gentle scrub with a soft brush may be helpful. Failure to remove all dirt from a wound predisposes to infection and may cause tattooing of the scar. Non-viable tissue is carefully removed with a scalpel.

TIMING OF WOUND CLOSURE

Wounds may be closed immediately by primary suture or at a later time by delayed primary suture. If the wound is fresh, clean and has little potential for infection, then it can be closed immediately. This is termed primary closure. If the wound is over 6 h old or obviously infected (e.g. as the result of a human or animal bite or if the wound has been made with an object used for cutting uncooked meat), then primary closure is out of the question as it will seal in the infecting organisms and lead to suppuration. Under these circumstances, the wound should not be closed immediately but it should be cleaned, inspected and a sterile dressing applied. Oral antibiotics should be given. The wound is then reinspected at 48 h and, if not infected at this time, it can be cleaned again and closed. This is known as delayed primary closure.

SURGICAL INSTRUMENTS REQUIRED FOR WOUND CLOSURE

Presterilized packs are available from the Sterile Services Unit of most hospitals and will contain all the instruments required to close minor wounds (Fig. 6.2). All that is required is found in a minor operations or small basic tray.

Sutures

Sutures are made of a variety of materials, both man-made and naturally occurring, and are either absorbed by the body or are non-absorbable. A range of sizes is also available and the material of the suture itself can be braided, twisted, monofilament or multi-filament, each with its own handling characteristics. The choice of which suture to use for a particular task is often, at first, bewildering.

Synthetic polymer materials are more biocompatible than natural materials, the latter of which evoke a greater tissue reaction. Monofilament sutures are smooth and run easily through tissues, whereas braided or twisted sutures generate more friction but have greater knot security. Generally, when suturing wounds of the skin, a synthetic monofilament suture is utilized and a double throw used in the first part of the knot to prevent slipping. If a surgical wound is closed with a subcuticular suture, then either absorbable or non-absorbable material may be used. The patient will have to return for the removal of a non-absorbable suture but the wound is secure as long as the suture remains, and less tissue reaction will result. Absorbable material used for subcuticular closure should be undyed to avoid tattooing of the scar. Some types of sutures, their characteristics (including times for complete absorption) and uses are given in Table 6.1.

Suture size appears complex. However, if a number appears on its own, then the larger the number, the thicker the suture (e.g. 2 Vicryl is thicker

TABLE 6.1 Common suture materials

MATERIAL	TRADE NAME	CHARACTERISTICS	COMMON USE
Polygactin 910	Vicryl	Absorbable (56–70 days) braided polymer	Subcuticular suture Deep wound suture Haemostatic tie
Catgut		Absorbable (90 days) twisted or monofilament made from sheep or ox intestine Much tissue reaction	Deep sutures in wounds
Polyglycolic acid	Dexon	Absorbable (60–90 days) braided multifilament polymer	Subcuticular suture Deep wound suture Haemostatic tie
Polydioxanone	PDS	Slowly absorbed (90–180 days) monofilament Little tissue reaction	Subcuticular suture
Silk		Braided non-absorbable multifilament from silkworm	Scalp suture
Polypropylene	Prolene	Synthetic non-absorbable monofilament	Skin suture

TABLE 6.2 Skin suture size by region

REGION	SUTURE SIZE	TIME UNTIL REMOVAL (DAYS)
Limbs	3/0 or 4/0	7
Trunk	3/0	7–10
Face	5/0 or 6/0	4–5
Scalp	0 or 2/0	5

than 1 Vicryl which is thicker than 0 Vicryl). If a size appears with a 0 (e.g. 2/0 Vicryl) then the larger the numerator, the finer the suture (e.g. 3/0 is finer than 2/0). The size of a suture used in a wound depends upon the wound site. The suture should not be removed too early or the wound will gape, nor should it be removed too late as the sutures will leave marks and become difficult and painful to remove. A general guide is given in Table 6.2.

Needles

Hand needles and those held by an instrument are in common use for skin suturing, but generally the use of hand needles should be discouraged because of the risk of needlestick injury. A curved needle held in a needle holder is most appropriate. The size of the needle required is related to the necessary calibre of the suture and the thickness of the skin. Smaller needles are used for delicate suturing and larger needles for suturing thicker skin such as the scalp. Cutting needles are needed to penetrate the skin. They are triangular in cross-section and the edges will cut through the skin. Curved needles with the third cutting edge on the convex side are known as reverse cutting needles and should be used in preference to cutting needles (which have the third cutting edge on the concave side of the needle and therefore towards the wound). The reverse cutting action makes it less easy for the suture to cut out of the wound.

Scalpels

Scalpels are available as a separate reusable handle with disposable blades or as a disposable ready-made-up scalpel (Fig. 6.2). Handles are of different sizes but a No. 3 handle is generally all that is needed as it accepts Nos 10, 11 and 15 blades. The No. 10 blade has a sharp point and is therefore used to make small stab incisions. The No. 15 blade has a small curved cutting edge and is useful for finer work. To avoid accidents, scalpel blades must never be mounted onto handles using the fingers. A needle holder is used to grasp the blade which is then slid onto the handle. When not in use, the scalpel should be placed in a receptacle, such as a sterile kidney dish, out of harm's way.

SURGICAL TECHNIQUE FOR WOUND CLOSURE

The aim of wound suture is to bring the correct layers of a wound together accurately without causing further damage. Tissues should be handled gently at all times. Forceps should also be used gently to avoid crushing the wound edges. Delicate toothed forceps (using the tooth as the wound-edge hook) are kinder to tissues than roughly used non-toothed forceps. The

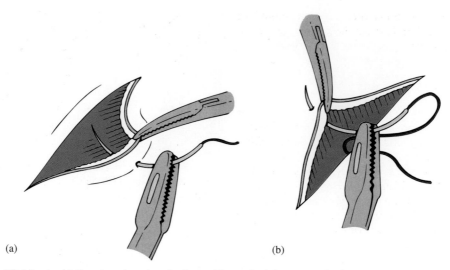

FIG 6.3   (a, b) Everting the wound edges with toothed forceps to facilitate insertion of the needle through the skin.

wound should be sutured only when clean and suturing should be performed in a well-lit sterile field. The technique is as follows:

- The needle is gripped by the needle holder, two thirds of the way along its length from the tip, usually at right angles to the shaft of the needle holder. The needle should enter the skin perpendicular to the surface and the bite should take at least the whole of the dermis (Fig. 6.3(a)). The needle is curved and this should be remembered when advancing it through tissues. The movement comes by supination of the forearm, not by pushing from the wrist.
- The temptation to pass the needle through both sides of the wound in the same bite should be resisted. This causes unequal thickness to be taken in on each bite leading to a step on the surface and dead space inside. Excessive force on the needle when trying to take bites which are too big will cause bending or snapping of the needle within the tissues.
- When the needle has been passed through one side of the wound, it is removed and an equal bite is taken from inside to out directly opposite. Again, the needle should enter perpendicularly and this is facilitated by lifting the wound edge gently with toothed forceps or a skin hook (Fig.6.3(b)).
- The suture is then tied. It is probably easiest for the occasional surgeon to perform instrument ties (Fig. 6.4). If a monofilament suture is used, then a double throw should be used initially to prevent slipping.
- The edges of the wound are apposed. Slight eversion of the edges is ideal; inversion or overlapping of the edges causes poor healing and a poor scar, as does undue eversion.
- Tension of the skin should be avoided. Sutures should not be tied so tightly that blanching of the skin occurs. This causes suture marks and may result

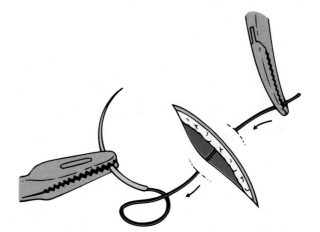

FIG 6.4   Performance of an instrument tie leaving a short end.

in the sutures cutting out. The subsequent swelling of the wound may also cause increased tension.
- All knots should be placed on one side of the wound. This will bring the edges into exact opposition.

Simple loop sutures, if inserted properly, will give an excellent cosmetic result in most cases. How long to leave sutures *in situ* depends on the speed of healing of that area of the body. A guide is given in Table 6.2.

PROBLEMS

Irregular wounds

Time should be taken to match the edges of irregular wounds to obtain good cosmesis. If two points can be seen to correspond then a suture should be inserted at that point. This will help to fit the rest of the 'jigsaw' together.

Wound tension

If the edges of the wound will not come together without tension, sutures should be inserted alternately at either end of the wound so that tension in the middle is gradually reduced. Mattress sutures can be used to diminish tension in the apposed edges. The edges can be advanced after undermining the skin with a scalpel or scissors. It is essential to avoid important nerves and vessels and not to devitalize skin. The correct layer to undermine in the face is just deep to the dermis. Blood supply is excellent and devitalization is unlikely. In the limbs and the trunk, undermining is best performed between the superficial and deep fascial layers. In the scalp, relaxing incisions along the undersurface of the galea, parallel to the wound, may be used. Haematoma is a common complication of any undermining.

Very long wounds

If sewn from one end, unequal bites lead to 'dog-earing'. The wound may be divided into more manageable lengths by placing a suture at the halfway point. Other sutures can be placed to further divide these halves if necessary.

Very deep wounds

Absorbable sutures may be placed deep in a wound (avoiding vital structures), inserted so that the knot is buried at the bottom. This will bring the skin edges closer together, reduce tension in the wound and obliterate dead space.

'Dog-ears'

If larger stitch intervals have been taken on one side of the wound than the other, a 'dog-ear' will be created. This heals poorly and is unsatisfactory cosmetically. A small 'dog-ear' can be dealt with by restitching at equal intervals on both sides. Larger 'dog-ears' must be removed by picking up the tip of the 'dog-ear' with a skin hook and excising the redundant skin. The resulting defect is then closed with sutures (Fig. 6.5).

Wounds of the lip, eyebrow and inside of the mouth

If a wound passes across the vermilion border of the lip or across the eyebrow, then great care must be

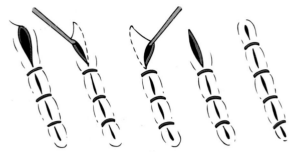

FIG 6.5 Removal of a 'dog-ear'. The tip of the 'dog-ear' is lifted with a skin hook and excised. The resultant defect is then resutured.

taken to suture accurately to avoid a step. This leads to a very unsightly result. Wounds inside the mouth need not be sutured unless a flap has been created which may accumulate food debris. If this is the case, then insertion of one or two absorbable sutures is required.

OTHER TECHNIQUES OF SKIN CLOSURE

Mattress suture

Bites are taken through the dermis as for a loop suture (described previously). The very edges of the wound are picked up by the suture so that the two ends are on the same side (Fig. 6.6). The suture is then tied. The deep and superficial bites ensure that tension is avoided and the edges are easily apposed and inversion avoided. This stitch causes slightly more tissue ischaemia than the simple loop suture and scarring is more prominent.

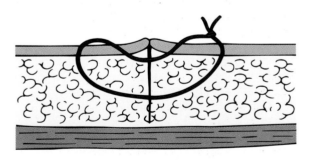

FIG 6.6 A mattress suture.

Continuous suture

The knot is tied so as to secure the first loop, and the suture is continued along the wound until the other end of the wound is reached and the second knot is tied (Fig. 6.7). Continuous loop or mattress sutures may be employed and the thread may be locked

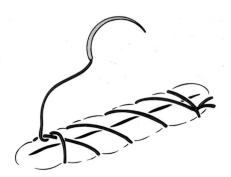

FIG 6.7   A simple continuous suture.

between each throw if desired (blanket stitch). Continuous sutures save time but bunching of the wound edges may be a problem for the inexperienced operator. More tissue strangulation is caused than with interrupted sutures and it is not generally advisable to close wounds at risk of infection in this way. The suture cannot always be partially removed to allow escape of pus.

Subcuticular suture

Equal bites of tissue are taken immediately beneath the surface of the skin on opposite sides of the wound from one end to the other, so that when the edges are drawn together the suture is not seen (Fig. 6.8). The ends may be secured by knots tied inside the wound, by beads on the skin surface or by knotting the two ends loosely in front of the wound; or there may be no knots, relying on the friction between suture and skin to keep the edges together. Absorbable materials (e.g. Vicryl or PDS) or non-

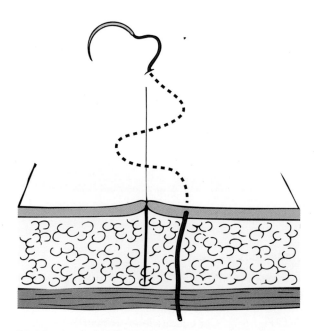

FIG 6.8   A subcuticular suture.

absorbable materials (e.g. Prolene) may be used. Non-absorbable subcuticular sutures are removed at a time appropriate for the region in which they are used. As with continuous sutures, subcuticular sutures should not be used in wounds at risk of being infected. With care, subcuticular suturing can give very pleasing cosmetic results and if absorbable sutures are used the patient need not attend for their removal.

Adhesive strips

Sterile adhesive tapes (Steri-strips) can be used to close superficial wounds which gape slightly, or as an adjunct to subcuticular closure. They should also be used to bring skin edges together in pretibial lacerations where the skin is often too thin for sutures to hold.

Clips

A variety of metal clips are available for skin closure. These can be inserted at the end of an operation at great speed and leave an acceptable cosmetic result. They do, however, cost considerably more than conventional sutures and require a special tool for removal.

Tissue glue

This is sometimes used to close minor wounds, particularly in children since its application is relatively atraumatic.

SAFETY ASPECTS

When suturing wounds, it is important to remember that the sharp points and blades used are contaminated by the patient's blood. This means that they are potentially vectors for transmission of blood-borne viruses. Intraoperative percutaneous injury has been shown to occur in 1.7–7% of operations performed. Those most at risk of injury are those who are most inexperienced in operating. Recommendations for precautions during wound closure and minor surgical procedures are:

- Impervious gloves should be worn. Double gloves are less often penetrated by a sharp.
- A gown that is impervious to water should be worn. In most gowns, there is a weak point where the cuffs join the sleeve. This should be covered by the cuff of the glove.
- Needles, blades and other 'sharps' should be placed in a dish when not being used. Sharp instruments should not be handed from one person to another. A receptacle containing the instrument should be used instead.

- Needles should never be resheathed. A high proportion of needlestick injuries occur in this way.
- All 'sharps' should be placed in a 'sharps' box at the end of a procedure.
- The finger should not be used as a guide for the needle and it is good practice to become accustomed to handling needles only with instruments and not with the fingers.
- Eye protection should be worn if blood and tissue aerosols are generated during a procedure or when operating on a high-risk patient.

7

Skin Biopsy

INTRODUCTION

Skin biopsy is a useful investigation for the diagnosis of cutaneous lesions or unusual rashes. Correct technique is essential, both in providing adequate material for histological diagnosis and in leaving the best cosmetic result for the patient.

INDICATIONS

Skin biopsy supplements clinical skills required for the diagnosis of cutaneous manifestations of systemic disease. Diagnosis and treatment of skin neoplasms can be undertaken. Tissue can be provided for micro-biology when unusual cutaneous infections are being considered, or for immunofluorescence when certain autoimmune disorders are suspected (Box 7.1).

However, biopsy of rashes often provides non-specific pathological changes, and should not be undertaken routinely. Referral to a dermatologist may circumvent the need to biopsy rashes or tumours. Surgical treatment of skin cancer should only be performed by those with specialist training.

TECHNIQUE

A step-by-step guide to skin biopsy is summarized in Box 7.2 and discussed below.

BOX 7.1   INDICATIONS FOR SKIN BIOPSY

Histological diagnosis (incision biopsy)
- Cutaneous changes in systemic disease (e.g. sarcoidosis, vasculitis, metastatic carcinoma or HIV-related Kaposi's sarcoma)
- Skin tumours prior to radiotherapy or definitive surgical treatment

Treatment (excision biopsy)
- Skin neoplasms (e.g. basal cell carcinoma or squamous cell carcinoma)

Diagnostic test
- e.g. Kveim test (sarcoidosis), direct immunofluorescence (autoimmune bullous disorders or systemic lupus erythematosus)

Fresh tissue for microbiology
- e.g. Cutaneous tuberculosis, opportunistic infections

BOX 7.2   STEP-BY-STEP GUIDE TO SKIN BIOPSY

- Explain the procedure fully to the patient and obtain signed consent form
- Check all equipment
  - sterile suture set
  - operating table and light
  - specimen pot with formalin
- Check the patient is not taking anticoagulant drugs or aspirin, and does not require antibiotic prophylaxis for valvular heart disease
- Lie the patient down
- Clean the area of skin, and mark the area to be excised with a skin-marker pen
- Inject local anaesthetic into the dermis
- Perform elliptical excision biopsy
- Close the defect with interrupted non-absorbable sutures
- Instruct the patient on wound care, and on date for suture removal

Explanation and preparation of the patient

Many patients are anxious about the procedure, and a few minutes of explanation can allay their fears. It is important to warn all patients about the risk of scarring. This should be clearly documented in the patient's notes. Certain body sites, such as joints or the back, tend to form stretched scars. Afro-Caribbean skin may produce keloids.

The patient is asked to sign a consent form. The procedure which is to be performed must be clearly stated. Enquiries are made about medication, particularly warfarin or aspirin, which interfere with haemostasis.

A brief medical history should be elicited. A check should be made for valvular heart disease as such patients should probably be given antibiotic prophylaxis. Current recommendations are listed in the British National Formulary.

Checking the equipment

If possible, the skin biopsy should be performed in a purpose-built minor operations theatre with an adjustable-height operating table. Cautery or diathermy equipment should be available for facial and scalp surgery. Nearby resuscitation equipment is mandatory.

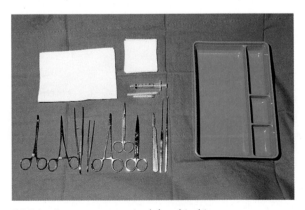

FIG 7.1   Instruments required for skin biopsy.

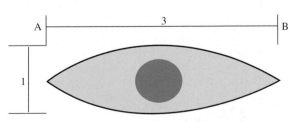

FIG 7.2   The longitudinal axis AB should follow the direction of relaxed skin lines. Failure to observe the '3:1' rule may result in puckered wound edges.

A complete suture set will be required (Fig. 7.1). This should include a scalpel with a No. 15 blade, skin hook, fine-toothed forceps, non-toothed forceps, stitch scissors, needle holder, swabs, syringe and needles. The specimen pot should contain 10% formal saline. Suture material is discussed in Chapter 6. Ideally, a trained nurse should be present.

Preparation for the biopsy

Positioning of the patient

The procedure is carried out with the patient lying down. The biopsy site should be stable and well illuminated.

Preparation of the surgeon

Hands should be washed twice in running water with 4% chlorhexidine (Hibiscrub) or 10% povidone-iodine (Betadine). Sterile disposable gloves should be worn. Masks and gowns are unnecessary, except when hepatitis C or HIV infection is suspected; goggles provide protection against splashing.

Local anaesthetic

Lignocaine or xylocaine (0.5–2%) with or without adrenaline (1/80 000 or 1/200 000) can be used for most procedures. Adrenaline provides a useful vasoconstrictor effect, but must not be used in areas supplied by end arteries, such as fingers, toes or penis, as intense vasospasm may lead to necrosis. EMLA cream (2.5% lignocaine, 2.5% prilocaine) applied to the biopsy site 1 h preoperatively induces variable anaesthesia; it is most effective on thin skin and in children. The maximum safe adult dose of lignocaine without adrenaline is 200 mg (or 3 mg/kg), for example 20 mL of 1% plain lignocaine. In children this dose is halved.

Performing an elliptical skin biopsy

The skin is cleaned with antiseptic solution or normal saline. The area to be removed is marked with a skin-marker pen; ball point or ink pens can lead to permanent tattooing of the scar. Alternatively, light scarification of the unanaesthetized skin with a No. 15 blade allows the incision lines to be planned without pain or risk of being washed off. The direction of the incision should fall within wrinkle lines, or relaxed tension lines. Skin is removed in an elliptical shape with a length to width ratio of 3:1 (Fig. 7.2). Circular defects can lead to 'dog-ear' formation.

The anaesthetic is injected with a small-gauge needle into the dermis. Successful technique results in the formation of a bleb around the injection site. If

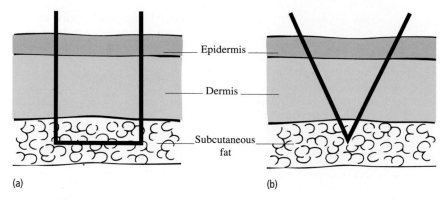

Epidermis

Dermis

Subcutaneous
fat

(a)   (b)

FIG 7.3   Schematic cross-section of biopsy site. (a) Correct and (b) incorrect angle of incision to achieve optimum apposition of wound edges.

adrenaline is used, blanching of the overlying skin should also occur. Attempts to inject large amounts of lignocaine into the subcutis are futile since this layer is relatively anaesthetic. Discomfort can be minimized by injecting slowly, warming the anaesthetic and using plain weak solutions.

The skin should be supported between finger and thumb, and, using the scalpel with the blade vertical to the skin, the marked ellipse is resected, including the full thickness of the skin. Inward-slanting incisions result in wedge-shaped inadequate specimens with unsatisfactory apposition of the wound edges (Fig. 7.3).

Holding the skin sample with skin hooks, or gently with forceps, the undersurface is freed with scalpel or scissors. The specimen is then placed in a correctly labelled formalin-containing pot. The accompanying request form must include the patient's details, a clinical summary and differential diagnosis to aid the pathologist.

Haemostasis is rarely a problem following firm pressure. The wound should be closed with interrupted non-absorbable sutures. However, not all defects require suturing; small wounds can be left to heal by secondary intention, with a hydrocolloid dressing.

POSTBIOPSY CARE

The patient should be warned to expect some local discomfort after a few hours. A dressing can be kept in place for 24–48 h; thereafter, the area can be gently cleaned. Dressings serve only to protect clothing from bloodstains. The date for suture removal will depend on the area biopsied. Certain sites, such as the lower leg, may result in tight wounds. Elevation or a knee-to-toe support bandage is then recommended.

The patient should be advised not to put undue tension on the area for at least 2 weeks after suture removal to prevent wound dehiscence.

SPECIALIZED BIOPSY TECHNIQUES

Punch biopsy

Disposable instruments with cutting metal cylinders between 3 and 6 mm diameter can be used to provide samples of skin for histological assessment. The area is prepared as described previously. With the skin under traction between thumb and finger, the instrument is pressed perpendicular to the skin and gently rotated. The specimen is gently lifted with fine forceps and cut at its base with scissors or scalpel (Fig. 7.4). The remaining defect can be either left open, cauterized, or sutured. Although this method is quicker, and is sometimes useful in children, better histological interpretation is achieved with the elliptical incision.

Shave biopsy

Prominent and superficial lesions, such as intradermal naevi or skin tags, can be removed by shaving the lesion flush to the skin surface with a scalpel. Haemostasis of the base can be achieved with direct pressure, cautery, or by the application of 20% aluminium chloride solution.

Curettage

A sharp-edged Volkmann spoon, and now disposable ring curettes, can be used to remove viral warts, seborrhoeic keratoses, cystic basal cell carcinomas and other superficial lesions. After anaesthetizing the area, the curette is held like a pen to scoop the lesion out of the skin. The fragmented sample must be sent for histological examination. The area is then cauterized. If removing malignant lesions, both steps are repeated at least twice, and only after expert tuition.

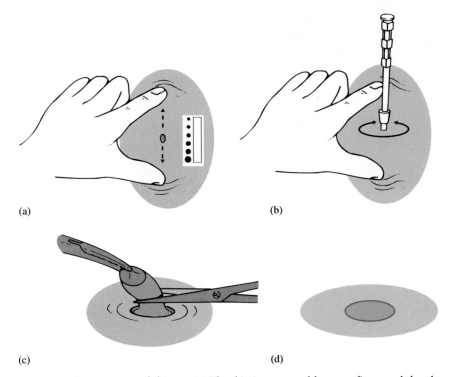

FIG 7.4 Performing a punch biopsy. (a) The skin is supported between finger and thumb. (b) The instrument is pushed downwards and gently rotated. (c) The core of tissue is removed by cutting at its base with scalpel or scissors (d) The remaining defect can be left open, cauterized or sutured.

Direct immunofluorescence

To aid the diagnosis of autoimmune skin disorders (e.g. pemphigoid, pemphigus, or systemic lupus erythematosus), a sample of skin can be studied for antibody and complement deposition. In the case of bullous disorders, a perilesional biopsy is necessary. The sample must *NOT* be put in formalin, but should be sent urgently to immunology, where it is usually stored in liquid nitrogen.

Kveim test

This is a useful confirmatory test for the diagnosis of sarcoidosis. Although insensitive, the test is relatively specific for its diagnosis. Kveim material is injected intradermally at a documented site. This can be adjacent to a naevus, and is preferably delineated by two or three microtattoos. A small-gauge needle is dipped in Indian ink, or sterile tattoo ink supplied by the hospital pharmacy, and then inserted into the skin. Permanent tattoo dots help identify the injection site, which is biopsied 4–6 weeks later. A granulomatous reaction supports the diagnosis of sarcoidosis, assuming the biopsy is clear of tattoo material.

COMPLICATIONS

Haemorrhage

Certain areas will bleed profusely, such as the face, scalp or fingers. Haemostasis is usually achieved after application of direct pressure, or wound closure. Rarely, small arteries may need to be ligated with absorbable suture.

Infection

The risk of infection is increased if poor aseptic technique is used, the wound is under tension or occlusive dressings are left unchanged. Good aftercare advice to the patient is essential. Local sepsis usually responds to topical antibiotics, but if there is evidence of cellulitis or lymphangitis, an oral antibiotic will be required.

Wound dehiscence

Wound breakdown can result from infection, excessive suture tension or poor technique. Resuturing is of no benefit following infection.

Keloid and poor scarring

The above factors, in addition to poor alignment of the wound, are also responsible for hypertrophic scars. Afro-Caribbean skin is prone to keloid formation. Poor scars are seen over sites of stretching, such as joints and the back.

8

Subcutaneous Hormone Implantation

INTRODUCTION

Hormone replacement therapy (HRT) is widely accepted for the treatment of menopausal symptoms, either during the climacteric or following surgical removal of the ovaries. The added protective benefits relating to osteoporosis and cardiovascular disease are being accepted by both doctors and patients. Furthermore, patient choice is being fostered and, where applicable, all routes of administration should be offered and tried so that ultimately the patient will determine which is best for her.

Implants have the advantage of excellent compliance and, between implant therapies, patients are not reminded daily of their medical conditions. Implants, both 17-beta-oestradiol and testosterone, are also valuable in treating patients with hypogonadism associated with hypopituitary disease.

INDICATIONS

By far the most common use of oestrogen implants is for routine HRT following hysterectomy and bilateral salpingo-oophorectomy. The initial implant may be inserted under the rectus sheath at the time of operation. Subsequent implants may be inserted when the implant wears out. Rarely, in a non-hysterectomized patient, when other routes may not prove satisfactory, the subcutaneous route may be used as a last resort. To protect the endometrium, regular intermittent progestogens should be supplemented (i.e. 1 mg norethisterone for the first 12 days of each calendar month), when a withdrawal bleed

may be expected. In the case where unopposed oestrogens are given, the endometrium should be monitored by ultrasound and endometrial biopsy from time to time. Testosterone implants are indicated when loss of libido occurs, particularly after hysterectomy and bilateral salpingo-oophorectomy. Implants are useful for patients who have hypopituitary function, particularly after surgical ablation.

PRELIMINARY CONSIDERATIONS

Dosage

A standard dose is 50 mg of 17-beta-oestradiol, which is usually repeated every 4–6 months. If the 50 mg dose does not control menopausal symptoms, then the implant may be increased to 100 mg. A 25 mg implant is also available. Testosterone is given at a dosage of 100 mg and this should last 4–6 months on average.

Procedure and future management

If the patient requires treatment at more frequent intervals, for example less than 6 months, then tachyphylaxis may occur; under these circumstances, an oestrogen examination should be made and implant therapy should be delayed until physiological levels have been attained. Severe symptoms may be relieved by the adjunct of oestrogen, either as a patch or orally.

TECHNIQUE

Equipment

A separate metal trocar and cannula are available for implanting the pellets (Fig. 8.1). This trocar, cannula and obturator are reusable. Hollow cannulae are difficult to clean thoroughly and central sterile department guidelines should be followed for clean-ing and resterilizing. To avoid the problem of reuse, a disposable plastic trocar and cannula (Fig. 8.1) is available, either singly or in a comprehensive pack (Fig. 8.2) which includes: swabs, syringe, needles, antiseptic, forceps, drapes, cotton wool balls, gloves, suture and a Band-Aid. If a pack is not used, all the individual components may be assembled prior to commencing the procedure. Local anaesthetic and the appropriate implant are all that is necessary to supplement the packs.

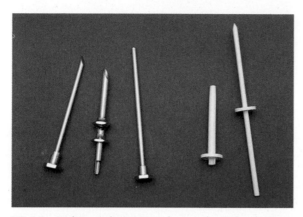

FIG 8.1 (Left) metal trocar and cannula with obturator (three pieces) and (right) plastic trocar and cannula with obturator (two pieces).

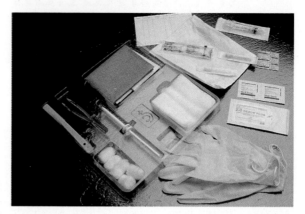

FIG 8.2 Pack ready for use.

Operational steps

1. The abdomen is swabbed with antiseptic.
2. Using a No. 1 needle, 5 mL of 1% lignocaine are injected into the lower abdomen, infiltrating a small area of skin, and then subcutaneously up to the hilt of the needle (Fig. 8.3).
3. The patient is draped.
4. A small incision is made into the skin.
5. The trocar and cannula are inserted as far as possible, along the direction of the local anaesthetic (Fig. 8.4).
6. The pellet is inserted into the cannula (Fig. 8.5).
7. The pellet is pushed down the cannula with the obturator (Fig. 8.6).
8. If two pellets are to be inserted, for example oestrogen and testosterone pellets, the cannula should be repositioned so that the two pellets do not lie adjacent to one another.
9. The cannula is removed.
10. The incision is sutured (or a Steri-strip is used if there is no bleeding).
11. A Band-Aid is placed over the wound (Fig. 8.7).

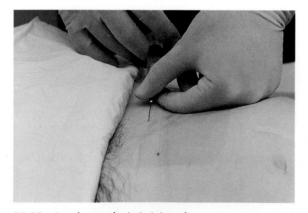

FIG 8.3 Local anaesthetic is injected.

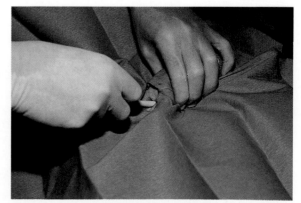

FIG 8.4 The trocar and cannula are inserted.

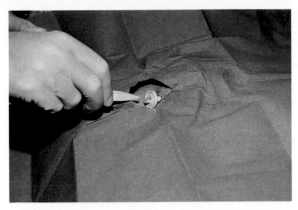

FIG 8.5   The pellet is inserted into the cannula.

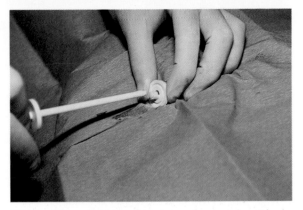

FIG 8.6   The pellet is pushed down the cannula with the obturator.

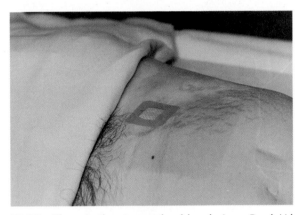

FIG 8.7   The procedure is completed by placing a Band-Aid over the wound.

Passage of a Nasogastric Tube

INTRODUCTION

The passage of a nasogastric tube is usually simple and innocuous. Nevertheless, patient discomfort can be reduced by sound technique and experience, which also minimize complications.

INDICATIONS

Nasogastric intubation is indicated for:

- aspiration of gastric contents for therapeutic or diagnostic purposes (i.e. after self-poisoning);
- enteric feeding;
- delivery of medication;
- assessment of upper gastrointestinal haemorrhage.

Preliminary considerations

The procedure is contraindicated in patients who have suffered recent fractures of the base of the skull. It is more hazardous in those who have suffered recent oesophageal trauma and in those with oesophageal strictures.

TECHNIQUE

Materials

Nasogastric tubes may be of the wide-calibre Ryle type or of finer bore (Figs 9.1 and 9.2). The former are more suitable for aspiration of stomach contents

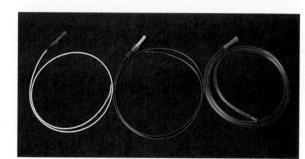

FIG 9.1 Polyvinyl chloride (red top) fine-bore (8 French gauge) nasogastric tube, polyurethane (blue top) fine-bore (8 French gauge) nasogastric tube, and Ryle's tube (16 French gauge).

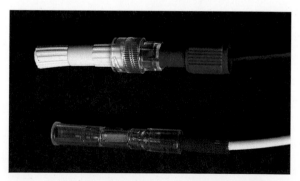

FIG 9.2 Guidewires and hubs from polyvinyl chloride (red top) and polyurethane (blue top) fine-bore tubes.

and gastric lavage, but are less comfortable for the patient and tend to cause oesophageal inflammation with the risk of haemorrhage and stricture. Fine-bore tubes are less irritant and are therefore preferred for long-term enteric feeding. There is now a wide range of such fine-bore tubes, with internal diameters typically of 1–1.5 mm. Polyurethane or polyvinyl chloride tubes are used commonly, the former being more resistant to kinking and allowing greater internal diameter for a given external tube diameter. This makes aspiration easier and allows the infusion of more viscous nutrients. The practice of attaching small weights to the distal end of fine-bore nasogastric tubes does not appear to reduce the rate of displacement from the stomach.

Insertion

Conscious patients should be told of the indications and should be given an explanation of the technique. Many patients find passage of a tube via the nasal cavity uncomfortable and a lignocaine spray can be applied locally. The length of tubing required is approximately equal to the distance from the ear lobe to the bridge of the nose to the xiphoid process. In conscious patients, intubation should be performed with the patient in the sitting position with the neck slightly flexed and clothing protected.

The tip of the Ryle's tube is lubricated with water-soluble material such as K-Y jelly. The guidewire of fine-bore tubes should be lubricated with tap water before insertion into the lumen of the tube to aid removal of the tube after placement (though some types are prelubricated).

The tube is then inserted slowly and horizontally along the floor of the nasal cavity (Fig. 9.3). When the distal end of the tube reaches the nasopharynx, the patient should be asked to swallow repeatedly as the tube is advanced. If necessary, this is helped by sips of water and rotation of the tube by the operator. Coughing, gagging or resistance to the passage of the tube may indicate misplacement; under these circumstances, the tube should be withdrawn before further attempts are made. In unconscious patients, nasogastric tubes, particularly of the fine-bore variety, may enter the trachea without adverse reactions. Passage of 50 cm of tube transnasally is usually sufficient to reach the stomach of an adult.

Confirmation that the tube is in the stomach

Confirmation of correct placement may be achieved by:

■ Aspiration of gastric contents and testing acidity with litmus paper. Even fine-bore tubes can be aspirated with a small syringe. Unfortunately, this method may be unreliable if gastric contents are aspirated from a tube misplaced in the airway after inhalation of gastric contents.
■ Blowing air down the nasogastric tube whilst listening over the epigastrium with a stethoscope. This method may also be unreliable as sounds may be transmitted from the lungs by a misplaced tube.
■ X-rays (Fig. 9.4). This is facilitated by a radio-opaque marker in the tube and is the most reliable method of confirming position. In conscious patients, the other methods usually suffice.

After confirming correct placement of the tube, it is secured to the nose or cheek by tape.

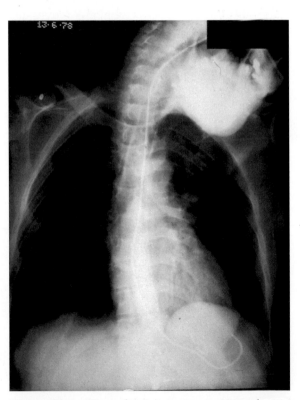

FIG 9.4 Chext X-ray showing correct position of nasogastric tube with the distal end in the stomach.

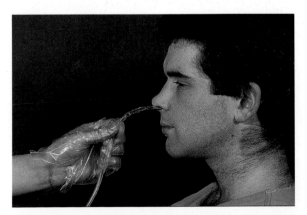

FIG 9.3 Passage of Ryle's tube in horizontal plane into nasal cavity of seated patient.

Difficulties of insertion and their circumvention

In the unconscious patient, the nasogastric tube can be guided into the oesophagus by two fingers at the back of the mouth. In patients with basal skull fractures (if the passage of a nasogastric tube is absolutely necessary), great care must be taken. Inserting a precurved nasopharyngeal tube, through which the nasogastric tube is passed, should avoid penetration of the retro-orbital space.

If the tube cannot be passed via the nasal cavity to the oropharynx at the first attempt, the other side of the nose should be used and/or a smaller tube substituted. In anaesthetized patients who are intubated endotracheally, difficulty in advancing the tube beyond the hypopharynx can be overcome by exerting gentle traction on the thyroid cartilage. Difficult intubations may require direct vision with a laryngoscope and the use of Magill forceps to guide the tube; in conscious patients, such a procedure requires sedation.

An alternative method that is now being used more commonly for difficult cases is passage of the tube under endoscopic guidance. In the rare event of an oesophageal stricture preventing insertion, endoscopic dilatation can be performed first. Fine-bore nasogastric tubes can be towed down alongside the endoscope, with the tip in the biopsy channel. Once in the stomach, the tip can be expelled from the endoscope by the passage of biopsy forceps and the endoscope carefully withdrawn. Alternatively, the fine-bore tubing can be passed down the biopsy channel. As the endoscope is withdrawn, the tube is advanced and kept in view. Subsequently, a nasopharyngeal tube is brought out through the mouth and used to tow the gastric tube out through the nose.

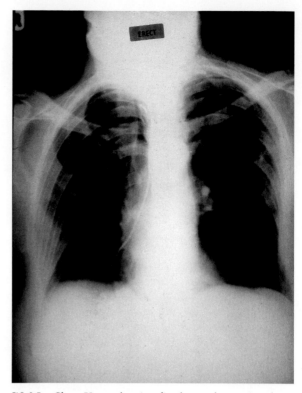

FIG 9.5   Chest X-ray showing fine-bore tube passing down the right main bronchus into the right lung.

COMPLICATIONS

Misplacement

Misplacement can occur in the following locations:

- *The cranial cavity*. This may occur when attempting to intubate patients who have suffered severe faciomaxillary trauma or basal skull fractures.
- *The respiratory tree* (Fig. 9.5). This may lead to pneumonia, pneumothorax, pulmonary haemorrhage, bronchopleural fistula, hydrothorax and empyema. Misplacement of nasogastric tubes is not prevented by endotracheal intubation as low-pressure cuffs may permit passage of tubes into the lungs.

Misplacement is sometimes signalled by difficulty in passage or withdrawal of the guidewire, although this is not invariably so. A partially withdrawn guidewire should not be reinserted without completely removing the nasogastric tube, as the wall of the tubing may be perforated by the more rigid guidewire.

Trauma

Insertion of a nasogastric tube can result in:

- epistaxis, pharyngeal or oesophageal perforation causing mediastinitis;
- gastric perforation.

Displacement of correctly inserted tubes

The following may occur:

- regurgitation into the oesophagus, especially after coughing and retching;
- aspiration of nasogastric feeds.

Oesophageal inflammation

Oesophageal inflammation leading to strictures can also occur.

FURTHER READING

Atkinson, M., Walford, S. and Allison, S.P. 1979: Endoscopic insertion of fine bore feeding tubes. *Lancet* **2**, 829–30.

Bastow, M.D. 1986: The complications of enteral nutrition. *Gut* **27** (Suppl. 1), 51–5.

Bouzarth, W.F. 1978: Intracranial nasogastric tube insertion. *Journal of Trauma* **18**, 818–19.

Mann, N.S., *et al.* 1984: Nasoenteral feeding tube insertion via fibreoptic endoscope for enteral hyperalimentation. *Journal of the American College of Nutrition* **3**, 333–9.

Perel, A., Ya'ari, Y. and Pizov, R. 1985: Forward displacement of the larynx for nasogastric tube insertion in intubated patients. *Critical Care Medicine* **13**, 204–5.

Silk, D.B.A. 1987: Towards the optimisation of enteral nutrition. *Clinical Nutrition* **6**, 61–74.

10

Proctoscopy, Sigmoidoscopy and Rectal Biopsy

INTRODUCTION

Proctoscopy, sigmoidoscopy and rectal biopsy form an essential part of the investigation of patients with lower gastrointestinal disease. The techniques can be performed easily in the out-patient clinic or at the bedside, and, in many cases, preceding bowel preparation is unnecessary. Techniques can be learnt easily by junior staff, and, when performed after adequate supervision and instruction, are safe and without significant discomfort for the patient.

INDICATIONS FOR PROCTOSIGMOIDOSCOPY

This is a mandatory investigation for patients whose history includes rectal bleeding, a change in bowel habit, or symptoms suggestive of local anorectal disease, such as the passage of mucus or perineal pain (Box 10.1). Because proctoscopy permits views of the distal rectum and anal canal only, it should always be accompanied by sigmoidoscopy.

The importance of sigmoidoscopy needs to be considered in the context that up to 40% of colorectal cancers occur in the distal 25 cm of the bowel. The use of flexible sigmoidoscopy will increase the yield still further, although the use of this instrument is not discussed here.

PREPARATION

This is a very embarrassing examination and it is essential to explain the procedure fully and to

BOX 10.1 INDICATIONS FOR PROCTOSIGMOIDOSCOPY

- Rectal bleeding
- Change in bowel habit
- Symptoms suggestive of colonic disease
- Anorectal disease
  — particularly haemorrhoids
- Anaemia
- Abdominal pain
- Chronic inflammatory bowel disease
  — diagnosis and assessment of response to treatment

reassure the patient. The procedure should not be unduly uncomfortable, but may cause crampy abdominal discomfort as air is being insufflated. This discomfort can be reduced by limiting the air insufflation to the smallest volume that ensures adequate visualization.

If a biopsy is to be taken, the examiner must make sure that the patient is not taking anticoagulant drugs or that he/she does not have a haemorrhagic diathesis. Patients with valvular heart disease or prosthetic valves need prophylactic antibiotics before the procedure. Current recommendations include amoxycillin (1 g intramuscularly) 1 h before the procedure, together with gentamicin (120 mg intravenously) immediately beforehand, followed by amoxycillin (500 mg orally) after 6 h. As an alternative, amoxycillin can be given intravenously at the same time as the gentamycin, followed by oral amoxycillin as before. For patients who are allergic to penicillin, vancomycin (1 g by slow intravenous infusion over 60 min) should be given, followed by gentamycin (120 mg intravenously) immediately beforehand.

TECHNIQUE

See Box 10.2.

BOX 10.2   STEP-BY-STEP GUIDE TO SIGMOIDOSCOPY

- Explain the procedure adequately to the patient
- Check all the equipment before starting the procedure; in particular
  — the light source to ensure that it is working
  — the air reservoir to ascertain that it does not leak
  — that a histology pot containing formalin is available
- Check that the patient is not taking warfarin or has a bleeding tendency, and that the patient does not have valvular heart disease (needing antibiotic prophylaxis)
- Position the patient to lie in the left lateral position
- Examine the anal region carefully (e.g. for piles, fissures and prolapse)
- Perform an initial digital rectal examination
- Perform proctoscopy, sigmoidoscopy and rectal biopsy
  — advance only when the lumen is visible; force must *not* be used
- Inform the patient about postprocedure rectal bleeding

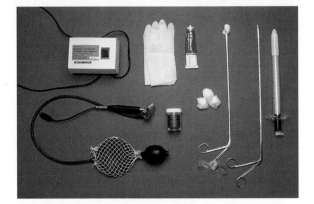

FIG 10.1   Essential equipment for sigmoidoscopy and rectal biopsy includes a suitable lubricant, disposable gloves, a sigmoidoscope, a light source, cotton wool pledgets, biopsy forceps and a histology pot containing formalin.

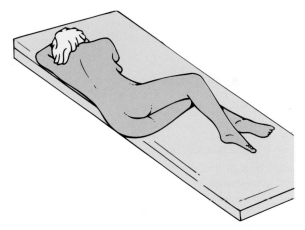

FIG 10.2   The ideal position for sigmoidoscopy involves the patient lying in the left lateral position with the buttocks over the edge of the couch.

Checking the equipment

The examiner should check that all the necessary equipment is available and in working order before starting the procedure (Fig. 10.1). Common problems are temperamental light sources and leaking air reservoirs. Disposable gloves should be worn and a little lubricating jelly applied to the patient's anus. 2% lignocaine is useful if local discomfort is anticipated. This might, for example, be the case for patients with anal Crohn's disease. Most hospitals now use disposable sigmoidoscopes (Welch–Allen) rather than the metal (Lloyd–Davies) sigmoidoscopes which need to be resterilized after use. A set of long biopsy forceps that can be passed through the sigmoidoscope is also necessary, together with pledgets of cotton wool to clear the sigmoidoscope should the view become obscured by faeces. The cotton wool is also useful to apply local pressure to the rectal mucosa in the event of troublesome postbiopsy bleeding. A specimen pot containing 10% formalin should be available for the biopsy.

Positioning the patient

The procedure is normally carried out with the patient in the left lateral position (Fig. 10.2). The buttocks need to be just over the edge of the couch, with the back relatively straight and a pillow under the head. The hips should be flexed to 90° but the patient should only partially flex the knees so that the lower legs are parallel to the edge of the couch. This ensures that the feet are well out of the way of the examiner's head! A blanket can be placed over the patient for warmth and modesty.

Perineal and digital rectal examination

Inspection of the perineum and a digital examination must precede proctosigmoidoscopy. The main reason for this is that a low rectal tumour may be missed

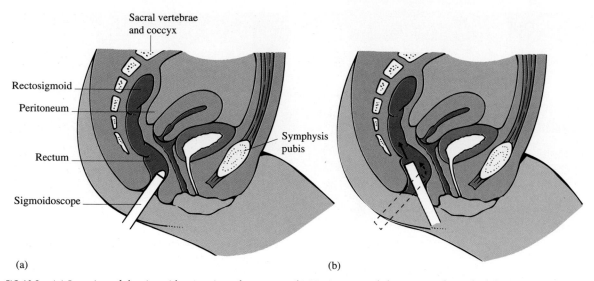

FIG 10.3   (a) Insertion of the sigmoidoscope into the rectum. (b) Having entered the rectum, the end of the instrument should be swung posteriorly and advanced under direct vision.

unless digital examination is performed. Inspection may reveal evidence of faecal soiling, pruritus ani, skin tags, external haemorrhoids, bulging or redness resulting from a perianal or ischiorectal abscess, fistulae or rectal prolapse. Digital examination with a well-lubricated finger will assess sphincter tone, tenderness or masses and, in males, the prostate size and consistency.

Proctosigmoidoscopy

An understanding of the anatomy is essential (Fig. 10.3). The method for insertion of the proctoscope is the same as that for sigmoidoscopy. Proctoscopy is particularly useful in assessing the severity of haemorrhoids and the presence of anal fissures.

The well-lubricated sigmoidoscope is inserted with steady pressure into the anal canal in the direction of the umbilicus; as the rectum is entered, the resistance will 'give'. At this point, the obturator should be removed and the light source connected to the sigmoidoscope. The tip of the instrument is then swung posteriorly under direct vision and advanced into the rectum, avoiding stool, or alternatively clearing the stool with cotton wool pledgets held in the long biopsy forceps.

If the rectum is loaded and it is impossible to see anything, then the procedure should be deferred until the patient has emptied the rectum – if necessary, following an enema or suppository.

The rectosigmoid junction is approximately 15 cm from the anal margin and here the lumen passes over the sacral promontory. Navigating the 'scope round the rectosigmoid junction can be difficult for the operator and uncomfortable for the patient. In some patients, it may be impossible to advance the instrument any further without anaesthesia. Negotiation of the rectosigmoid junction should not be regarded as a challenge if it is difficult! A more experienced person should be asked for help where necessary.

During the passage of the sigmoidoscope, sufficient air to open the lumen ahead is all that is necessary. Overenthusiastic insufflation will make the procedure very uncomfortable for the patient; it is worth remembering that the pressure in the air reservoir bulb is the same as that within the lumen of the rectum. The sigmoidoscope should be advanced only when the way ahead is visible. *Force must never be used.* This is particularly important when examining patients with ulcerative colitis where the mucosa is very friable; excessive force or insufflation may perforate the bowel wall. Potential problems encountered during the procedure are listed in Box 10.3.

Having reached the limit of the examination, the colour of the stool should be noted. If it is streaked with blood, this implies proximal disease. The instrument is then carefully withdrawn, looking for evidence of mucosal abnormality, polyps or carcinoma. It is on the way down that the formal examination takes place.

Normal rectal mucosa has a smooth, glistening pink appearance, through which the vascular pattern is clearly visible (Fig. 10.4). Mucosal changes that occur in inflammatory bowel disease include granularity, hyperaemia and contact bleeding. with more severe inflammation, pus and blood may be present in the lumen, together with active ulceration. Haemorrhoids appear as cherry-like protuberances in the anal canal and may show signs of recent bleeding.

BOX 10.3   PROBLEMS THAT MAY OCCUR DURING SIGMOIDOSCOPY

Problem
- Procedure is too painful for the patient

- View is obscured by faeces

- Excessive postbiopsy bleeding

- Perforation

Advice
- Consider anal fissure or abscess collection
- Try using lignocaine gel
  — if unsuccessful, postpone the procedure

- Use cotton wool pledgets through the sigmoido-scope to clear the view
- Repeat the procedure after the patient has evacu-ated the bowels following a suppository or enema

- Apply pressure with cotton wool pledgets
- Warn the patient that they may notice some rectal bleeding
  — if excessive, admit patient for observation and check clotting factors

- Risk is reduced by taking the biopsy postero-laterally and hence extraperitoneally
- Barium enemas should NOT be performed within 5 days of rectal biopsy
- Admit the patient for surgical review

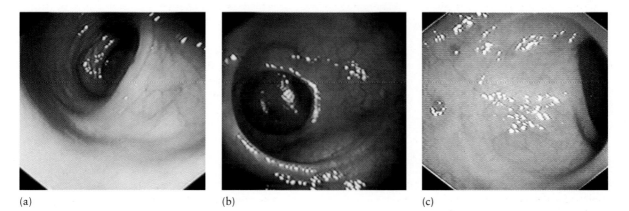

(a)   (b)   (c)

FIG 10.4   Normal rectal mucosa: (a) viewed towards the rectosigmoid junction; (b) viewed approaching the rectosigmoid junction; (c) viewed at the rectosigmoid junction.

Rectal biopsy

Even if the rectal mucosa looks normal, it is still useful to perform a rectal biopsy. This is particularly true for patients with diarrhoea where histology may reveal granulomata typical of Crohn's disease. It is safer to take biopsies from the extraperitoneal portion of the rectum; that is, posterolaterally within about 8–10 cm from the anal verge. The window attachment of the sigmoidoscope is removed and the biopsy forceps are passed through. With the window open, the distended bowel collapses. Under direct vision, an adequate portion of mucosa is biopsied by rotating the forceps with the jaws closed together and the application of gentle traction to detach the sample.

Following the biopsy, the mucosa must be inspected for signs of excessive bleeding; if necessary, cotton wool attached to forceps can be used to apply pressure to the bleeding mucosa. The patient must be told to expect some bleeding with the next bowel action.

After rectal biopsy, at least 5 days should be allowed to elapse before a barium enema examina-tion is performed. This is because the breach of the mucosa at biopsy may form the site of a perforation due to the high intrarectal pressure of a subsequent enema.

CONCLUSIONS

All patients with symptoms suggestive of lower gastrointestinal pathology, including a change in bowel habit with weight loss, should undergo proctosigmoidoscopy. Even if the rectal mucosa looks normal, a biopsy should be performed as this may reveal granulomata typical of Crohn's disease.

Proctosigmoidoscopy, when performed properly, is safe and easy and can be performed in either a clinic or surgery.

FURTHER READING

Endocarditis Working Party. British Society for Antimicrobial Chemotherapy. 1990: *Lancet* 335, 88–9.

11

Percutaneous Liver Biopsy

INTRODUCTION

The removal of a sample of liver tissue for laboratory investigation provides valuable and often diagnostic information about liver disease and many systemic illnesses. There are several approaches to liver biopsy: percutaneous, transjugular, laparoscopic or at laparotomy. The percutaneous approach is adequate for most routine medical purposes and is the approach described in this chapter. In recent years, targeted biopsy with imaging, usually ultrasonic, has become obligatory for focal lesions. Indeed, some would argue that blind percutaneous biopsy, which has been utilized since the late 1940s, is now outdated and that all liver biopsies, whether for focal or diffuse disease, should be performed with imaging. Nevertheless, in the UK, blind biopsy has been shown to be no more hazardous than biopsy with imaging and is still widely used (Gilmore *et al.*, 1995). Indeed, in many hospitals in less-developed countries, blind biopsy is still the only technique available. Although the trend is clearly towards more biopsies under ultrasound control, both blind and targeted biopsy methods are described here as the management and complications are largely the same.

INDICATIONS

Liver biopsy is commonly used to establish a diagnosis of cirrhosis, as well as to identify specific causes of chronic liver disease and responses to treatment (e.g. chronic hepatitis B/C and interferon therapy). The diagnosis of primary or secondary tumours in the liver can be confirmed histologically. In dealing with possible primary liver tumours, consideration must be given to subsequent curative resection, but the potential risks of disseminating malignancy with biopsy have probably been exaggerated (Wright, 1989). These risks include the possibility of introducing malignant cells into the bloodstream and the growth of tumour along the needle track.

BOX 11.1   INDICATIONS FOR LIVER BIOPSY

Primary liver disease
- Acute liver dysfunction
- Chronic hepatitis (for diagnosis and treatment)
- Cirrhosis
- Unexplained jaundice

Unexplained hepatomegaly or hepatosplenomegaly
- Sarcoidosis
- Amyloidosis

Drug effects
- For diagnosis or monitoring therapy (e.g. methotrexate in psoriasis)

Screening for familial disease
- Haemochromatosis
- Wilson's disease
- Alpha-1-antitrypsin deficiency

Assessment following liver transplantation

Malignancy
- Primary liver tumours (see text)
- Secondary carcinoma or carcinoid
- Staging of lymphoma

PRELIMINARY CONSIDERATIONS

All invasive investigations can cause morbidity and even mortality; liver biopsy is no exception. Reviews of large series have shown an incidence of major complications in 0.32% of cases (Terry, 1952) and mortality rates of between 0.015 and 0.33% (Gilmore et al., 1995; McGill et al., 1990; Terry, 1952; Zamcheck and Klausenstock, 1953). The critical question is whether the value of the information obtained outweighs the risks.

A check-list of important preliminary investigations and procedures is shown in Box 11.2, and the important points are discussed below.

BOX 11.2 PRELIMINARY CONSIDERATIONS FOR LIVER BIOPSY

- Fitness for biopsy
- Informed consent of patient
- Cooperation of patient
  — ability to hold breath
  — ability to lie flat
- Ultrasound scan of liver (to exclude dilated ducts and to target lesions). Many now scan patients at time of biopsy
- Potential 'anatomical barriers'
  — ascites
  — skin infection
  — right lung consolidation
  — pleural effusion
- Haematology
  — international normalized ratio (INR) <1.3
  — haemoglobin >10 g/dL
  — platelet count >80 × 10^9/L
- Check bleeding time in high-risk patients

Consent and cooperation

As with all invasive procedures, a signed consent form is required after appropriate explanations about the biopsy and the risks involved. This needs particular sensitivity with liver biopsy as a brash approach may well terrify the patient. Full cooperation is essential as the patient must hold his/her breath in expiration, an apparently simple task which some find particularly difficult. In children, a general anaesthetic is usually required.

CONTRAINDICATIONS

Because the patient has to lie flat and breath-hold for a few seconds, liver biopsy is contraindicated in patients with cardiac and/or respiratory failure. Pneumothorax is always a potential hazard with blind biopsy through the classical route in the eighth space in the mid-axillary line.

The anatomical pathway to the liver should be free from pathology such as skin infection, pleural

effusion or ascites. In itself, ascites is not an absolute contraindication but it makes the procedure technically more difficult and the risk of bleeding is greater. Empyema and subphrenic abscess are absolute contraindications to biopsy, and puncture of hydatid cysts may precipitate anaphylactic reactions. Preoperative ultrasound examination should prevent needling a dilated and obstructed biliary tract, and occasionally the gall-bladder may be punctured during blind biopsies.

Haematological contraindications

Any bleeding tendency constitutes a relative contraindication to liver biopsy. Traditionally, it has been considered safe to perform a biopsy when the INR is less than 1.3 and the platelet count is greater than 80 × 10^9/L. Unfortunately, serious and sometimes fatal bleeding may occur when these parameters are normal. When there are doubts about potential bleeding on other grounds, such as impaired liver function, undue spontaneous bruising or an elevated bilirubin level, the bleeding time should also be checked.

If the INR is greater than 1.3, the procedure should be postponed and Vitamin K_1 (10 mg) given slowly intravenously on a daily basis until the INR is within the normal range. If the INR does not fall to 1.3 or below after 3 days, and biopsy is considered essential, the procedure should be covered with an infusion of fresh frozen plasma (1 unit in the hour preceding biopsy and 1 unit in the following hour). An alternative approach under these circumstances would be to be to perform a transjugular biopsy, but this technique requires highly specialized skills.

Thrombocytopenia is less of a hazard in liver biopsy, although if the platelet count is less than 80 × 10^9/L, and the biopsy is considered essential, platelet concentrate should be used.

In all cases, the patient's blood group should be known and serum saved. If the blood group is unusual, compatible blood must be immediately available.

TECHNIQUE

The three techniques in blind biopsy, involving the Menghini, Surecut (modified Menghini) and Trucut needles, utilize a common approach. Following careful explanation of the procedure and after obtaining a signed consent form, the patient is placed supine, close to and parallel to the edge of the bed. The right arm is abducted (Fig. 11.1). The patient's chest is percussed over the right hemithorax in the mid-axillary line, and the intercostal space (which lies immediately below the cephalic limit of hepatic

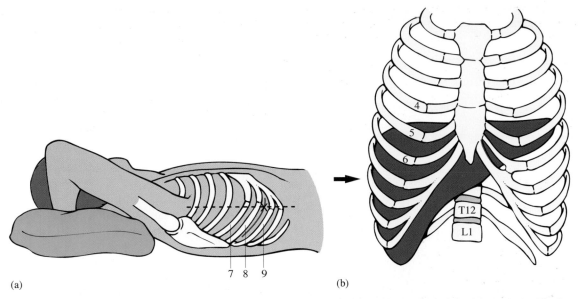

(a)   (b)

FIG 11.1   (a) The position of the patient for liver biopsy. The oblique red line indicates the eighth rib interspace. The intersection of this line with the mid-axillary line is indicated and marks a suitable site for biopsy in the majority of patients. (b) The surface marking of the liver showing site of biopsy in the eighth intercostal space.

dullness on full expiration) is marked; in most patients, this is the eighth space in the mid-axillary line. Use of this site provides an ample depth of liver for puncture. The use of ultrasound obviates the need for these manoeuvres. If the liver is grossly enlarged, a subcostal approach may be adopted.

Sedation is not usually necessary and indeed is better avoided as the patient's full cooperation is required. The skin is cleansed with antiseptic and the biopsy site demarcated with sterile towels. Using a 25 G needle, the skin just above the rib is anaesthetized with 2–3 mL of 1% lignocaine. Then, using a 21 G needle, the deeper tissues of the chest wall are infiltrated with local anaesthetic. The liver capsule can be anaesthetized by injection of 0.5–1.0 mL of lignocaine directly into the superficial liver substance with the patient holding his/her breath in expiration. Whilst the anaesthetic is taking effect, the patient can be taught how to inhale and exhale deeply and how to hold their breath on deep expiration. It is critical that the patient understands this step. Once the patient has mastered this, the skin over the biopsy site is nicked with a sharp scalpel.

Menghini technique

The Menghini needle (Fig. 11.2) is available in three diameters: 1.0, 1.4 and 1.8 mm. The 1.4 mm needle is used routinely for adults. The tip of the needle is oblique and has a cutting edge. A small nail with a flattened head sits in the base of the needle, preventing aspiration of the biopsy into the syringe. A triangular-based nail with a sharp point is often provided

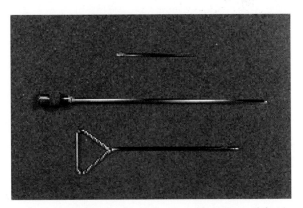

FIG 11.2   Menghini needle. From top to bottom: nail fitting in the base of the needle; the Menghini needle which is attached to a 10–20 mL syringe; and a triangular-based nail supplied in most packs to bore through the skin.

with the kits to puncture the skin and intercostal muscles. We prefer to do this with a fine scalpel. A little saline is drawn into a 10 or 20 mL syringe which is attached to the Menghini needle. The biopsy needle is then advanced through the puncture site into the intercostal muscles, but not yet into the liver itself, thus minimizing the risk of tearing the liver as the patient breathes.

A little saline is then expelled through the needle to extrude any subcutaneous debris. With the patient holding their breath in *expiration*, steady continuous suction is applied to the syringe, and the needle is then quickly inserted into and withdrawn from the liver.

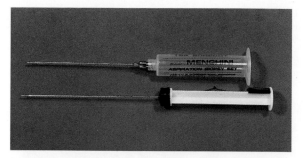

(a)

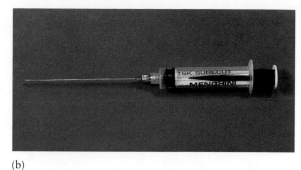

(b)

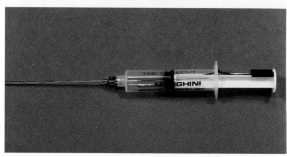

(c)

FIG 11.3 The Surecut system. (a) The two components. (b) The system ready for insertion through the skin with the point projecting from the cutting biopsy needle. (c) The plunger withdrawn to the stop on the plastic guard ready for insertion into the liver.

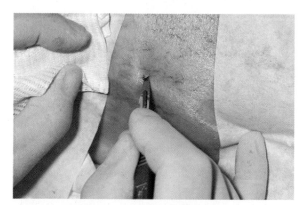

(a)

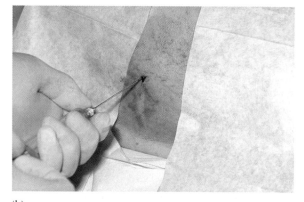

(b)

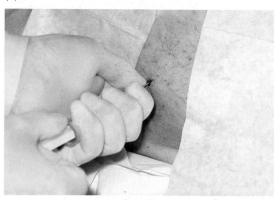

(c)

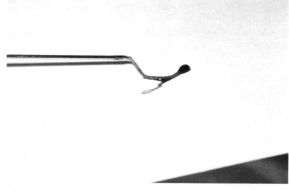

(d)

FIG 11.4 Use of the Surecut system. (a) The skin is nicked with a scalpel; no attempt should be made to bore through the skin with the needle itself. (b) With the plunger depressed and the barrel of the syringe held in the operator's left hand, the end of the needle is inserted in the intercostal muscles; at this stage, the patient is asked to breathe out. (c) With the patient breath-holding in expiration, the plunger is withdrawn to the notch on the guard and the needle is inserted into the liver substance. (d) With the plunger still held out and the patient still breath-holding in expiration, the needle is withdrawn and the biopsy is extruded onto a card.

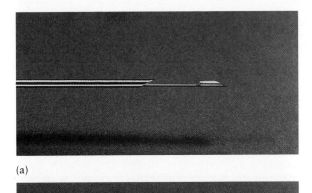

(a)

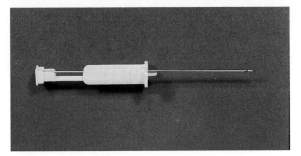

(b)

(c)

FIG 11.5   Trucut system. (a) The end of the needle with the inner trocar advanced to show the notch into which the biopsy is taken. (b) The needle in the close position. (c) The needle with the trocar advanced to show the notch.

Many pathologists prefer the specimen to be extruded onto a piece of white card to prevent fragmentation. At this stage, tissue that is required for special treatment, such as electron microscopy, culture or immunology, can be removed, and the remainder placed immediately into 10% buffered formalin for standard histopathological examination.

The Surecut technique

The Surecut biopsy needle (Fig. 11.3) works on a similar principle to that of the Menghini needle. It consists of a disposable unit with a short trocar which is connected to the plunger of the syringe and which occludes the biopsy needle (Fig. 11.3(a)). With the plunger down, the sharp point of the trocar just protrudes from the end of the cutting biopsy needle (Fig. 11.3(b)). With the plunger withdrawn (Fig. 11.3(c)), the distal 2–3 cm of the needle is available to receive the biopsy. Two sizes of needle are available: 1.4 and 1.8 mm in diameter; the 1.4 mm type is suitable for most liver biopsies.

Using a similar approach to that described above, the skin is nicked with a fine scalpel (Fig. 11.4(a)). There is no need to penetrate any deeper at this stage. The needle is then inserted, with plunger down, through the nick in the skin (Fig. 11.4(b)) and then into the intercostal muscles, but no deeper. For the next step, in a right-handed operator, the barrel of the syringe is conveniently held in the operator's left hand and the plunger held with the finger and thumb of the right hand. The patient is asked to breathe out,

the plunger is withdrawn to the stop on the plastic guard, and the biopsy needle is inserted into the liver substance (Fig. 11.4(c)). The whole unit is then withdrawn with the plunger still out, and the biopsy is extruded (Fig. 11.4(d)).

Trucut technique

This method is difficult to master and involves a different type of instrument (Fig. 11.5). The inner trocar of the Trucut needle has a notch, which is exposed as the trocar is advanced (Fig. 11.5(a)).

With the notch closed (Fig. 11.5(b)), the needle is advanced slowly 2–3 cm into the liver, with the patient breath-holding in expiration. Whilst holding the outer sheath, the operator advances the inner trocar further into the liver substance to expose the notch (Fig. 11.5(c)). The outer sheath is then advanced to cut off the biopsy, which is retained in the notch, and the needle is withdrawn.

Choice of biopsy technique

We prefer the Surecut method because it is simple, easy to use and good biopsies are obtained with the new, sharp needles. The needle is ideal for use by those learning liver biopsy. With very hard cirrhotic livers, the Trucut needle provides larger, less-fragmented samples, but the method requires much practice and confidence. Whereas the Menghini and Surecut techniques require the needle to be in the liver for no more than 1 s, even the slickest operator needs to have the Trucut needle within the liver substance for at least 3 or 4 s for a good biopsy.

Targeted liver biopsy under radiological control

The use of ultrasound has revolutionized liver biopsy, which is now used in many parts of the developed world, being increasingly performed by interventional radiologists. This technique is obligatory for biopsying focal lesions such as secondary carcinomatous and carcinoid tumours. A number of special biopsy guns are available, such as the Temno gun (Fig. 11.6), with which it should be possible to obtain material from lesions as small as 1 cm in diameter. The use of these biopsy guns should be restricted to interventional radiologists.

Many argue the case for ultrasonic visualization of the liver before and/or at the time of biopsy. Certainly, there is much to be said for this technique when dealing with shrunken cirrhotic livers and livers of unusual shape.

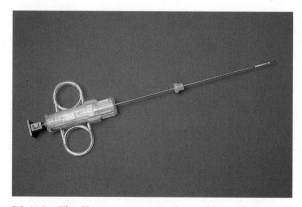

FIG 11.6 The Temno automatic disposable guillotine soft tissue needle. This needle acts using the Trucut technique. It is spring loaded and, upon firing, the sample is trapped in the sample notch.

POSTBIOPSY CARE

Following biopsy, the skin is cleaned and the puncture site is covered with a plaster. Much care is needed when dealing with patients who have had biopsies and are known to be hepatitis B or C positive. Patients are often more comfortable lying on the right side for 2 h after biopsy. They should remain in bed for 8 h and then be gently mobilized. Pulse, temperature and blood pressure should be recorded half-hourly for 2 h, and then hourly for 6 h.

Where biopsies are carried out in radiological departments, it is critical that patients are accompanied and monitored by experienced staff at all times. Disasters have occurred when postbiopsy patients have been left unsupervised in corridors while awaiting return to the wards.

We perform liver biopsies in the first half of the morning, and retain the patient in hospital until the following morning. Others perform liver biopsies on a day-case basis, allowing discharge after 4–6 h if the clinical state permits, provided the patient stays within reach of the hospital overnight and is given a telephone number by which to contact a member of hospital staff in the event of adverse reactions (Box 11.3).

BOX 11.3   COMPLICATIONS OF LIVER BIOPSY

Vasovagal episodes (usually within a few seconds or minutes)
Pain
— at the biopsy site
— right hypochondrium
— right shoulder
Pneumothorax
Bleeding
— intra-abdominal
— pleural (rare)
Biliary peritonitis
Septicaemia (may occur if the patient has unsuspected cholangitis)

Failure to obtain tissue

Inexperienced or nervous operators often fail to obtain tissue because they do not puncture the liver; a firm confident thrust is required to penetrate the liver, particularly if it is cirrhotic. Other failures may occur with faulty positioning of obese patients, or in patients with small cirrhotic livers, when identification of hepatic dullness may prove difficult or misleading. Biopsy with ultrasound control is essential under these circumstances.

COMPLICATIONS

The earliest complication, which may occur within the first minute after liver biopsy, is a vasovagal attack. This is alarming because the patient becomes pale, sweaty and hypotensive and may lose consciousness. To the inexperienced, this may simulate a sudden severe bleed. Recovery quickly ensues and is encouraged by raising the foot of the bed. The commonest reaction is pain, which usually reflects the wearing off of local anaesthesia and is reduced by simple analgesia. Often, there is some referred shoulder pain during or after biopsy. Localized discomfort in the right upper quadrant may indicate subcapsular accumulation of blood.

Fortunately, significant haemorrhage following biopsy is rare. When it happens, it usually occurs within the first few hours after the biopsy. Fatal haemorrhage has occurred from parenchymal tears, when the patient breathes or coughs whilst the needle is within the liver, or as a result of perforation of distended portal or hepatic veins or aberrant arteries. Bleeding into the pleural cavity is exceptionally rare and is believed to be due to damage to the intercostal vessels. Such damage may be avoided by keeping the biopsy needle close to the upper border of the rib. Progressive deterioration of the patient, in spite of transfusion, and continuing evidence of bleeding requires laparotomy, after a review of the patient's haemostatic mechanisms.

Small pneumothoraces caused by the needle nicking the pleural reflection are probably more common than is realized. However, they rarely require treatment. A rare but potentially fatal complication is peritonitis following perforation of the bowel or of an infected, dilated biliary system. Should fever and rigors follow a biopsy, blood cultures should be taken and the patient started on high doses of antibiotics. It may be necessary to seek surgical help in order to initiate decompression of the biliary system.

REFERENCES

Gilmore, I.T., Burroughs, A., Murray-Lyon, I. M., Williams, R., Jenkins, D. and Hopkins, A. 1995: Indications, methods, and outcomes of percutaneous liver biopsy in England and Wales: an audit by the British Society of Gastroenterology and the Royal College of Physicians of London. *Gut* **33**, 437–41.

McGill, D.B., Rarela, J., Zinmeister, A.R. and Ott, B.J. 1990: A 21 year experience with major haemorrhage after percutaneous liver biopsy. *Gastroenterology* **99**, 1396–1400.

Terry, R. 1952: Risks of needle biopsy of the liver. *British Medical Journal* **1**, 1102–5.

Wright, T. 1989: Cancer of the liver. *Current Opinions in Gastroenterology* **5**, 405–10.

Zamcheck, N. and Klausenstock, O. 1953: Liver biopsy (concluded): the risk of needle biopsy. *New England Journal of Medicine* **249**, 1062–9.

12

Abdominal Paracentesis

INTRODUCTION

Removal of ascitic fluid, abdominal paracentesis, is useful for diagnostic purposes and has important therapeutic applications. In the UK and North America, cirrhosis of the liver is the commonest cause of ascites but there are many other causes which are listed in Box 12.1. Some patients with cirrhosis requiring paracentesis may be of high-risk infective status and appropriate precautions need to be taken with invasive procedures (*see* Chapter 1).

INDICATIONS

Diagnostic

A small-volume (20–50 mL) diagnostic paracentesis should be part of the routine initial examination of any patient with ascites. This is particularly important because of the high risk of spontaneous bacterial peritonitis (SPB) in cirrhotic patients. It may also be useful in the diagnosis of the acute surgical abdomen.

Therapeutic

Relief of symptoms

In patients with abdominal malignancy, as with carcinoma of the ovary, removal of tense ascites may be necessary to relieve painful abdominal distension and/or distressing breathlessness.

BOX 12.1   CAUSES OF ASCITES

Associated with chronic diseases
- Cirrhosis of the liver[a]
- Heart failure[a]
- Abdominal malignancy[a]
- Liver disease without cirrhosis
- Hepatic vein occlusion
- Constrictive pericarditis
- Polyserositis (e.g. systemic lupus erythematosus)
- Nephrotic syndrome
- Infections (e.g. tuberculosis)
- Pancreatitis

Associated with acute abdomen
- Trauma (haemoperitoneum)
- Bacterial peritonitis
- Acute pancreatitis

[a]Common causes.

Control of hepatic ascites

In many centres, therapeutic paracentesis, used in association with plasma expanders, is the initial treatment for patients with tense or moderate ascites. This is because the rate of reaccumulation of ascites, the length of hospital stay and the financial costs are more favourable with paracentesis than with diuretics alone (Kyriacou and Hayes, 1995).

DIAGNOSTIC PARACENTESIS

CONTRAINDICATIONS

There are virtually none. Bleeding dyscrasias render the procedure more hazardous (*see* Chapter 11) but, in any case, most patients with hepatic ascites will have some degree of coagulopathy. Fortunately, the small size of the diagnostic needle (19 G) makes significant bleeding unlikely.

TECHNIQUE

First, the patient should be checked to ensure that the bladder is empty. The site chosen should avoid distended superficial veins, the inferior epigastric vessels (see below) and sites of previous surgery. The spleen must be avoided if it is enlarged. Usually, a point in the flank, within the U-shaped area of ascitic dullness, is suitable.

For a simple diagnostic aspiration, little preparation is required and the procedure can be performed in the out-patient clinic or surgery. The operator should wear gloves but gowns and drapes are unnecessary. The selected site should be cleaned with antiseptic and the skin and deeper tissues down to the peritoneum anaesthetized with 1% lignocaine. It may be helpful to roll the patient from the supine position towards the side of the aspiration with smaller volumes of ascites. For most diagnostic aspirations, a 20 mL syringe with a 19 G needle is appropriate. Gentle suction is applied to the plunger whilst the needle is advanced through the abdominal wall. As the peritoneum is pierced there is usually a distinct 'give', with reflux of ascitic fluid into the barrel of the syringe. If the aspiration is truly diagnostic, samples are sent to the microbiology, cytology and chemical pathology laboratories (Table 12.1). The visual appearance of ascitic fluid may point to its aetiology. Most fluids are straw coloured but turbidity suggests bacterial infection. Bloodstained fluids may indicate malignancy, and milky ascitic fluid usually indicates lymphatic obstruction due to malignancy.

If the patient is a known cirrhotic and the aspiration has been undertaken to exclude SPB, then cell counts and microbiological examinations are all that are required. Inoculation of ascitic fluid into blood culture bottles improves the sensitivity over conventional methods of culture (Runyon, 1994).

THERAPEUTIC LARGE-VOLUME PARACENTESIS

PRECAUTIONS AND CONTRAINDICATIONS

The removal of large volumes of ascitic fluid (> 5 L) is obviously associated with more hazards than simple diagnostic paracentesis. This is particularly so when the paracentesis is being performed therapeutically for ascites in cirrhosis. Care must be taken in patients with bleeding dyscrasias related to underlying liver disease, and the comments made in Chapter 11 apply also to paracentesis. A normal international normalized ratio (INR) and normal platelet count does not necessarily prevent excessive bleeding.

The dangers of rapid removal of large volumes of ascites have probably been overstressed in the past but, particularly in cirrhosis, paracenteses may induce

TABLE 12.1 Useful tests on ascitic fluid

LABORATORY	TEST AND CLINICAL SIGNIFICANCE
Microbiology	Gram stain of centrifuged deposit[a] Culture (including tuberculosis) and inoculation of blood culture bottles[a]
Cytology	White cell count (>250/mL suggests infection)[a] Examination for malignant cells
Chemical pathology	Level of pH 7.34 or less associated with SBP Ascitic fluid total protein (AFTP) usually <25 g/L in uncomplicated cirrhosis, but not reliable Serum-ascites gradient correlates well with portal pressure[b] Ascitic amylase level always very high in acute pancreatitis Gamma GT elevated in hepatoma

[a]Essential investigation when spontaneous bacterial peritonitis is suspected.
[b]The serum-ascites albumin gradient is calculated by subtracting the ascitic albumin concentration from the serum albumin concentration. Patients with gradients >11 g/L have portal hypertension.

hypovolaemia, hypotension, renal failure, and hepatic encephalopathy.

Premedication is rarely necessary for paracentesis and, in particular, should be avoided when liver disease is present or suspected, because of the risk of precipitating encephalopathy.

TECHNIQUE

For this procedure, aseptic technique is required with mask, gloves, gown and drapes. In 'high-risk' patients, the operator needs protection too! As with diagnostic paracentesis, the patient's bladder should be empty. A check should be made to ensure that all the required equipment is available (Box 12.2). It is particularly irritating to find that, after the catheter has been inserted, there are no adaptors to connect up with the drainage apparatus.

The site chosen for the insertion of the catheter should be well away from abdominal scars, dilated superficial veins and the inferior epigastric vessels. We prefer using a site in the flank within the area of ascitic dullness between the anterior part of the iliac crest and the umbilicus (Fig. 12.1). Alternatively, a site may be chosen in the midline between the umbilicus and the symphysis pubis, caudal to the upper limit of ascitic dullness. If the cannula is inserted in the flank, it will pass through skin, superficial and deep fascia, the aponeurosis or muscle of the external oblique, the internal oblique muscle, the transversus abdominis muscle, the fascia transversalis and extraperitoneal fat before entering the peritoneal cavity. If the midline is selected, the muscle layers will be replaced by the virtually bloodless linea alba. Where there is doubt, ultrasound examination can be used to identify the most suitable site.

After swabbing the skin with antiseptic, local anaesthesia is induced with 1% lignocaine. The skin is then nicked with a small scalpel blade, and a peritoneal catheter and stylet (Fig. 12.2) are inserted through the skin and subcutaneous tissues into the peritoneal cavity. This is best done using a boring movement with the catheter gripped like a pen. The 'give' on entering the peritoneal cavity is characteristic and the operator's grip on the distal end of the catheter prevents any uncontrolled plunge into the depths of the peritoneal cavity. The archaic metal trocars and cannulae that are still offered for paracentesis by some hospitals should not be used.

Once the catheter is in the peritoneal cavity, the

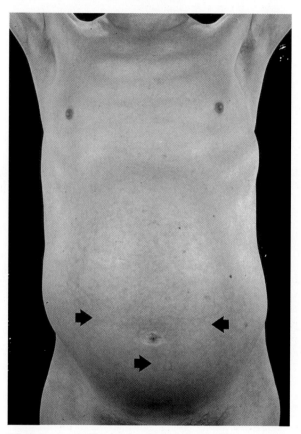

FIG 12.1 A suitable site for the insertion of the paracentesis catheter, in this patient with ascites, is between the umbilicus and the anterior superior iliac spine.

BOX 12.2 EQUIPMENT REQUIRED FOR LARGE-VOLUME PARACENTESIS

■ 10 mL 1% lignocaine
■ 25 G (orange-hubbed) needle
■ 21 G (green-hubbed) needle
■ Surgical blade
■ Peritoneal dialysis catheter and drainage tubes
■ Catheter drainage bag
■ Antiseptic wash (e.g. Betadine)
■ Suture (e.g. 3/0 silk)
■ Sterile needle holder and scissors
■ Suitable adaptors

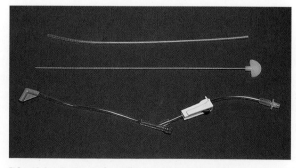

FIG 12.2 Peritoneal catheter apparatus. From top to bottom: the catheter, trocar, adaptor tubing and clamp to control flow. Before starting, appropriate adaptors should be placed at hand to connect with the drainage bag.

stylet can be withdrawn 1–2 cm to create a flexible end. The catheter is then directed inferiorly, posteriorly and, if necessary, laterally, into the right or left paracolic gutters. At this stage, the stylet is removed and samples are taken for the laboratory. The catheter is then connected to the drainage tubes which, in turn, are attached to a closed drainage bag. Many hospitals use a urinary catheter drainage bag for this purpose. There are no strict guidelines as to the rate of drainage of ascites but 3 L over a 4 h period is reasonable. Large-volume paracenteses have been performed more quickly without clinical disturbances.

In patients with cirrhosis, recurrent large-volume therapeutic paracenteses are more safely performed concurrently with administration of plasma expanders. There is good evidence that this reduces the incidence of hypovolaemia, renal failure and encephalopathy (Gines and Arroyo, 1993). The most effective plasma expander for this procedure is salt-free albumin at a dosage of 6–8 g intravenously for each litre of ascitic fluid removed. It has been suggested that cirrhotic patients with peripheral oedema can safely undergo paracentesis without using concurrent plasma expanders (Kyriacou and Hayes, 1995).

What to do if the catheter stops draining

It is not unusual for the catheter to stop draining when clinically there is still residual ascites. First, the catheter should be checked to ensure it has not been pulled out! However, failure to drain is most likely due to fibrinous exudate or omentum around the distal end of the catheter. If this is so, withdrawal by 2 or 3 cm or rotation of the catheter may re-establish flow. Alternatively, turning the patient onto the side of drainage may help.

If simple measures on the ward are unsuccessful, a radiologist should be asked to perform ultrasound and, if necessary, to reposition the tube. Where there are adhesions and/or loculation of ascites, there may be no alternative but to reinsert the catheter on the opposite side.

AFTERCARE

After the ascites has been drained as effectively as possible, a small amount of ascitic fluid will continue to leak through the puncture site for 2 or 3 days. The application of a colostomy bag to collect the fluid is a less messy way of dealing with this than wads of absorbent cotton wool. Continuing diuretic therapy is obligatory after paracentesis in cirrhotic patients.

BOX 12.3 COMPLICATIONS OF LARGE VOLUME ABDOMINAL PARACENTESIS

Local
- Bleeding
- Infection of abdominal wall
- Bacterial peritonitis
- Perforation of gut or bladder

General
- Hypovolaemia
- Hypotension
- Renal failure
- Portosystemic encephalopathy

COMPLICATIONS

Local and general complications of abdominal paracentesis are listed in Box 12.3. The problems of hypovolaemia, hypotension and renal failure have been discussed earlier.

Bacterial peritonitis (causing fever, tachycardia and abdominal pain after 24–48 h) is not an unusual complication in patients with cirrhosis. The draining fluid will become turbid but routine sampling for microbiological culture should avoid delay in diagnosis.

Significant haemorrhage from the abdominal wall is rare, being recorded in 0.9% of all paracenteses in one series (Runyon, 1986).

Bowel or bladder perforation are rare complications. Local adhesions following previous intra-abdominal sepsis or surgery make this more likely, hence the need to avoid such sites for the paracentesis. Direct puncture of the bowel is usually self-evident with faeculent drainage through the catheter. If this unusual complication occurs, the patient should be started on broad-spectrum antibiotics and observed carefully in hospital. Surgical advice should be sought, but unless there is deterioration a laparotomy is not necessary.

REFERENCES

Gines, P. and Arroyo, V. 1993: Paracentesis in the management of cirrhotic ascites. *Journal of Hepatology* **17** (Suppl. 2), S14–18.

Kyriacou, K. and Hayes, P. 1995: Managing the patient with hepatic ascites. *Hospital Update* July 316–21.

Runyon, B.A. 1986: Paracentesis of ascitic fluid. *Archives of Internal Medicine* **146**, 2259–61.

Runyon, B.A. 1994: Care of patients with ascites. *New England Journal of Medicine* **330**, 337–42.

13

Urethral and Suprapubic Catheterization

INTRODUCTION

Catheterization of the urinary bladder is an everyday procedure carried out by doctors of all specialities. Urethral catheterization is still the commonest technique although the suprapubic route is becoming increasingly popular.

URETHRAL CATHETERIZATION

INDICATIONS

The commonest indications for urethral catheterization (Box 13.1) are urinary retention and/or incontinence. A catheter may also be required for postoperative drainage to monitor output, to give treatment, or as part of an investigation of the urinary tract.

CONTRAINDICATIONS

There are, arguably, no absolute contraindications to urethral catheterization. However, a history of pelvic or perineal trauma associated with perineal bruising and swelling and/or blood at the meatus calls for extreme caution. Ideally, a urological opinion should be sought. A history of urethral strictures or false passages may be elicited and signal caution; in this

BOX 13.1   INDICATIONS FOR URETHRAL CATHETERIZATION

Retention
— acute
— chronic
Incontinence
— intractable problem, resistant to treatment
— patient unfit for definitive treatment
To maintain bladder drainage following surgery (e.g. prostatectomy or cystoplasty)
Monitoring urine output
To give treatment (e.g. intravesical chemotherapy or prolonged bladder distension)
Investigations (e.g. cystometry or micturating cystourethrography)

case, the procedure may be carried out with care, but should be stopped if difficulties are encountered.

TECHNIQUE OF MALE URETHRAL CATHETERIZATION

Preparing the patient

A relaxed patient is essential if the catheter is to be passed successfully. The patient should be positioned supine with the legs relaxed and flat on the bed. Flexed hips and drawn up knees, even if minimal, are sure signs of an anxious patient and a contracting impassable sphincter.

Choice of catheter

Most male catheterizations are for retention of urine and/or incontinence, and a 'two-way' catheter is appropriate. In order to minimize complications, the ideal catheter should be made of an inert material and have a negligible calibre and balloon diameter. Silicone catheters are not totally inert but cause less irritative reaction than the common latex rubber catheter. As a rough guide, a silicone catheter may be left *in situ* for 3 months but a rubber catheter should be changed after 3 weeks. Rubber catheters are much cheaper and are perfectly satisfactory for short-term use. Silicone-coated rubber catheters are not suitable for long-term use as the coating may 'peel off' and expose the rubber beneath. A small calibre is desirable since this minimizes urethral trauma and the inevitable urethritis. However, if it is too small the drainage will be inadequate; 16 F is a reasonable compromise. The balloon can cause intense irritation and should be designed to hold no more than 10 mL of water.

Catheters with a third channel that allows for bladder irrigation are used widely in the management of clot retention, and after prostate and bladder surgery.

Technique

Most hospitals supply a 'catheterization pack' containing the essentials to carry out the procedure. Catheterization should be carried out as cleanly as possible but all drainage systems will become contaminated eventually. The penis is cleansed with a non-irritant antiseptic (Fig. 13.1(a)) and pulled through a hole in a sterile paper towel to provide a sterile field. Lignocaine jelly (15 mL, 0.5%) is squeezed down the urethra with one hand while holding the penis with the other (Fig. 13.1(b)). After introduction of the lubricant (the jelly will only provide anaesthesia if at least 10 min are allowed to elapse before proceeding), it is massaged gently down the urethra towards the perineum (Fig. 13.1(c)).

Pulling the penis gently upward to straighten out the urethra, pressure on the glans is released and the catheter is introduced into the meatus in the line of the urethra (Fig. 13.1(d)). There should be no need to handle the catheter. 'No touch' sterility can be maintained by using sterile forceps (often supplied in the catheterization pack) or by using the inner wrapper of the catheter pack.

Generally, the catheter will pass easily down the penile and bulbar urethra but a slight resistance is often felt as it passes through the posterior urethra. At this stage, the patient will usually complain of some slight discomfort in his bottom. Once past this point, the catheter will slip in very easily.

There may be some immediate backflow of urine but one should continue to pass the catheter until the side arm reaches the meatus. Only then can one be reasonably certain that the catheter is in the bladder (Fig. 13.1(e)). It is possible for the eye of the catheter to lie within the bladder while the balloon remains within the prostatic urethra (Fig. 13.2). The balloon should be inflated with no more than 10 mL of water. Urine may not appear immediately – the jelly often blocks the catheter; a small squirt of water will clear it easily (Fig. 13.3). The catheter is then connected to a closed drainage bag and the residual volume noted – this is very often useful to the urologist and/or nephrologist (Fig. 13.4).

Occasionally, one will be confident that the catheter has entered the bladder but despite clearing the lumen there is little or no urine. The diagnosis of acute retention may be 'obvious' but one should beware of the oliguric or anuric man with an acute abdomen posing as acute retention. It is not a rare event for the on-call urologist to admit patients with small bowel obstruction, diverticular disease or leaking abdominal aneurisms!

Getting stuck

The usual causes of failure to pass the catheter are phimosis, urethral stricture, an occluding prostate or, most commonly, a tense patient. *A catheter introducer should never be used* unless specific training has been received; help should be sought from a more experienced colleague. If the catheter will not pass, then the suprapubic route is an alternative but this should be avoided in the presence of undiagnosed haematuria. If one is really stuck, the pain of acute retention can be quickly relieved by aspirating 200 mL of urine from just above the symphasis pubis with a large syringe and needle, provided that the bladder is palpable.

Letting down the bladder

It is still occasionally taught that the bladder should be decompressed slowly after catheterization for chronic retention, namely that 500 mL aliquots should be run off with a period of catheter clamping between each. It was thought that this would prevent sudden falls in intravesical pressure which would cause massive haemorrhage. There is no rationale for this since the removal of very small volumes will dramatically reduce intravesical pressure. Indeed, failure to adequately drain the bladder is a positive disadvantage since this increases the chance of infection.

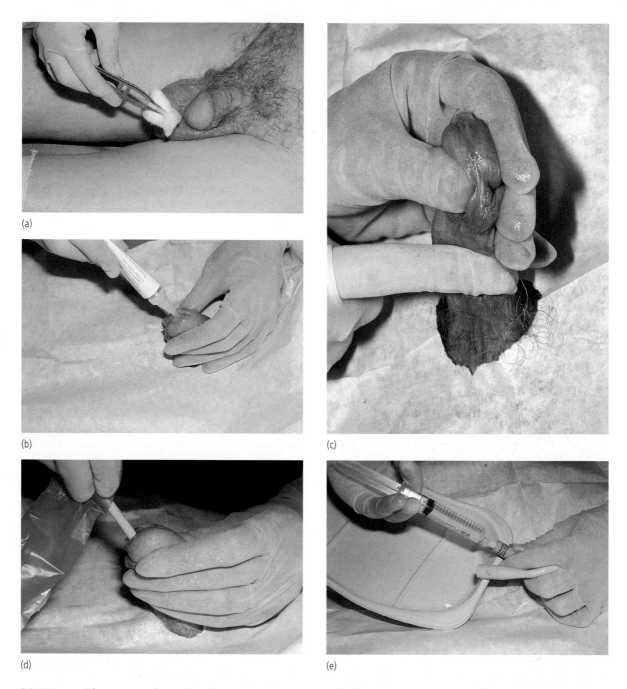

FIG 13.1 (a) The penis is cleansed with non-irritant antiseptic. (b) Lignocaine jelly (15 ml, 0.5%) is squeezed down the urethra with one hand, while holding the penis with the other. (c) The meatus is gently squeezed to prevent the jelly from leaking out and then it is massaged down the urethra towards the perineum. (d) Pulling the penis gently upward, in order to straighten out the urethra, the pressure on the glans is released and the catheter is introduced into the meatus in the line of the urethra. (e) The catheter continues to be passed until the side arm reaches the meatus. The balloon is inflated with no more than 10 ml of water.

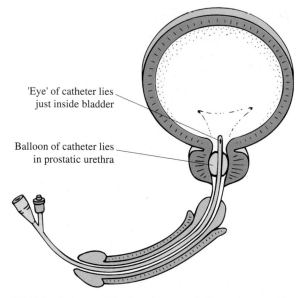

'Eye' of catheter lies just inside bladder

Balloon of catheter lies in prostatic urethra

FIG 13.2 It is possible for the eye of the catheter to lie within the bladder while the balloon remains within the prostatic urethra. A backflow or urine will occur but inflation of the balloon will be extremely painful.

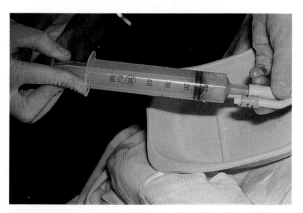

FIG 13.3 The lubricating jelly often blocks the catheter. A small squirt of saline or water from a bladder syringe will clear it easily.

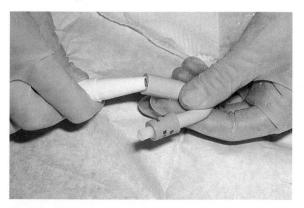

FIG 13.4 The catheter is connected to a closed drainage bag and the residual volume is noted.

FEMALE URETHRAL CATHETERIZATION

The female urethra is much shorter and relatively less difficult to catheterize. Again, proper positioning of a relaxed patient is vital: the knees must be adequately flexed and abducted. The urethral meatus may be obvious, but in older postmenopausal women the meatus may well retreat into the vagina. Occasionally, the urethra will be stenosed and dilation or a suprapubic catheter may be required.

SUPRAPUBIC CATHETERIZATION

INDICATIONS AND ADVANTAGES

The commonest indications for suprapubic catheterization (Box 13.2) are urinary retention and long-term drainage for incontinence. A suprapubic catheter may also be used for postoperative drainage (perhaps in addition to a urethral catheter), following various urological procedures including bladder neck suspension, culposuspension, cystoplasty and bladder substitution: it ensures adequate urinary drainage and facilitates trials of voiding. It is particularly useful in the management of urethral trauma (Box 13.3).

The bladder is usually palpable in both acute and chronic retention, so suprapubic catheterization should be straightforward. With care, insertion of the catheter should not be any more uncomfortable than the passage of a urethral catheter, and, once in place, the suprapubic catheter is generally much more

BOX 13.2 INDICATIONS FOR SUPRAPUBIC CATHETERIZATION

- Urinary retention
- Long-term catheterization for incontinence
- Postoperative urinary drainage
- Urethral trauma

BOX 13.3 ADVANTAGES OF SUPRAPUBIC CATHETERIZATION

- No urethral trauma or catheter-induced urethritis
- Greater patient comfort
- Enables continuous irrigation at transurethral resection of prostate
- Facilitates trial of voiding
- Very easy to change catheter

acceptable. The urethra is not traumatized and urethritis cannot occur. Finally, most men suffering retention will come to transurethral prostatectomy; the suprapubic catheter facilitates both continuous irrigation during the procedure and trials of voiding.

Long-term catheterization of the female bladder can present particular problems, especially in the presence of neuropathy (e.g. when multiple sclerosis causes incontinence). The urethral orifice in women is a perineal structure and the catheter (because they are forced to sit on it) will be a constant source of irritation. Patients are often unable to reposition themselves or the catheter and the catheter balloon tends to exert continuous traction on the bladder neck and urethra. In addition, the neuropathic bladder is often hypercontractile and persistently seeks to expel the catheter. The net result may well be complete erosion of the bladder neck and urethra. Men are not immune to this type of complication and complete erosion of the penile urethra is not unknown in paraplegics.

A suprapubic catheter is valuable in the immediate management of urethral trauma. Its insertion requires no great urological expertise and it often provides simple, adequate urinary drainage in a severely injured patient.

DIFFICULTIES AND CONTRAINDICATIONS

It is absolutely imperative to aspirate urine from the proposed site of catheterization (Box 13.4). Failure to aspirate urine with a needle is an absolute contraindication to continue! The other major contraindication is the presence of undiagnosed haematuria; there is risk of seeding transitional cell carcinoma along the catheter track.

Although changing an established suprapubic catheter is in many ways easier than changing a urethral catheter, the new catheter must be inserted

BOX 13.4 CONTRAINDICATIONS TO SUPRAPUBIC CATHETERIZATION, AND POSSIBLE DIFFICULTIES

Contraindications
■ Inability to aspirate urine
■ Undiagnosed haematuria

Difficulties
■ When changing the catheter, the new catheter must be inserted immediately to avoid closure of track
■ Catheterization of the neuropathic bladder may require general anaesthesia

immediately. Even a short delay will allow the criss-crossing muscle fibres of the detrusor to contract and obliterate the track.

Neuropathic bladders are often hyper-reflexic and cannot be filled sufficiently to allow straightforward suprapubic catheterization; a general anaesthetic is usually required.

TECHNIQUE OF SUPRAPUBIC CATHETERIZATION

Various types of suprapubic introducers and catheters are available. This chapter will describe the Lawrence introducer (Fig. 13.5), which has several advantages: it is easy to use with a local anaesthetic, it enables the use of self-retaining balloon catheters (no sutures required), and it is relatively inexpensive. The principles for the successful use of other introducers are the same. The 'catheterization pack' supplied by most hospitals will contain most of the other essentials, but a disposable scalpel or scalpel blade will also be required.

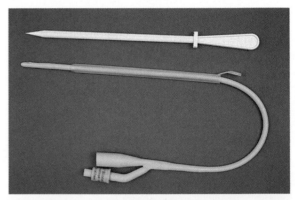
(a)

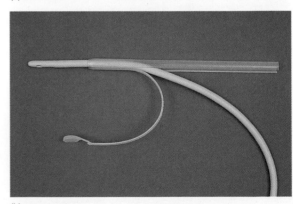
(b)

FIG 13.5 (a) The Lawrence introducer for a suprapubic urinary catheter has two components: (top) a sharpened trocar and (bottom) a plastic sheath with a tear-off strip. (b) The tear-off strip which releases the sheath after placement of the catheter (see text)

Preparing the patient

A relaxed and confident patient is essential if the catheter is to be placed successfully. It may be necessary to shave a few square centimetres of skin just above the centre of the symphysis pubis.

Choice of catheter

The 'ideal' urinary catheter has been described earlier. The Lawrence introducer is available in three sizes and is designed for use with a 10, 12 or 16 French-gauge catheter.

Technique

A check is made to ensure that the bladder can be palpated and a point 2–4 cm above the symphysis pubis is selected. Every effort should be made to carry out the procedure as cleanly as possible, although all drainage systems will become contaminated eventually. At least 20 mL of 1% lignocaine is drawn up and a weal raised in the skin at the selected site with an orange-hubbed 23 G needle. The area is cleaned with a non-irritant antiseptic and paper towels used to provide a sterile field. A green-hubbed 21 G needle is then used and advanced into the anaesthetized area, expelling anaesthetic as one proceeds, taking great care to keep needle and syringe perpendicular to the surface of the couch (Fig. 13.6).

Reaching the bladder wall

If the distension of the bladder has been correctly assessed, and if there is not too much adipose tissue, the bladder wall will be reached quite easily. At this point, the patient will often complain of increased discomfort and it is important to infiltrate the area well. At least 20 mL of the lignocaine solution should be used to infiltrate the intended catheter track. There may be a slight 'give' as the needle enters the bladder and one should then be able to aspirate clear urine. *The procedure must not be continued unless urine has been aspirated.*

The scalpel blade is used to make a 1 cm incision in the skin. It is important to carry this incision through the fat, fascia and almost to the bladder wall. The patient must be warned that they will feel pressure but no pain. Using the same line taken by the needle, the introducer is pushed firmly using a twisting motion, with the operator's other hand guarding against a sudden plunge into the bladder. If the tissues have been properly anaesthetized there will be no pain, but there may be discomfort on an already overfull bladder. The introducer will suddenly 'give' as it enters the bladder.

Before proceeding, the correct size of catheter (connected to an appropriate drainage bag) is placed

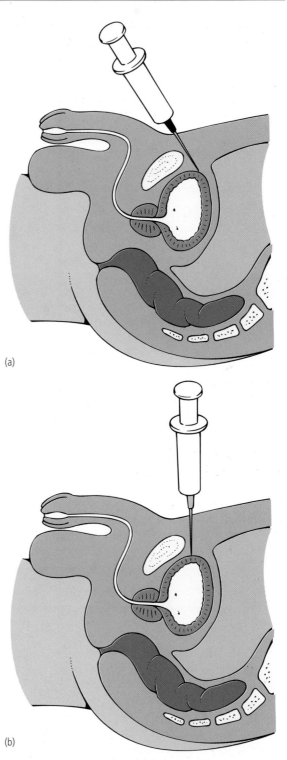

(a)

(b)

FIG 13.6   (a) The tendency to keep the needle at an angle to the patient's abdomen should be avoided. (b) The track of the needle should be perpendicular to the couch.

at hand, with the means to inflate the retaining balloon. The trocar is removed with the right hand, taking care to prevent the sheath from coming out by using the left hand. As the trocar is removed, urine will gush from the sheath, often under considerable pressure. The flow is staunched with a finger and then the full length of the catheter is fed down the sheath. The retaining balloon should be immediately filled – if the bladder is allowed to empty, it may 'slip off' the catheter as it deflates. The sheath is pulled out along the catheter and the tear-off strip pulled away to remove it. The puncture site may require a simple dressing at first if there is some bleeding, but dressings are not usually necessary after 24 h. The residual volume is noted.

Getting stuck

If urine cannot be aspirated, the procedure *must be stopped* and help sought. Perhaps this is not a bladder in retention; the diagnosis should be reconsidered. An ultrasound examination will usually clinch things if the physical signs are equivocal. Sometimes, excess adipose tissue prevents a green-hubbed needle from reaching the bladder – a longer one should be cautiously tried. The line of the needle should be checked to make sure it is correct; one must remember to keep needle and syringe perpendicular to the couch – if anything, pointed slightly downward towards the pelvis. If insertion of the introducer causes pain, then more anaesthetic is required. One must be aware that in women with

bladder neck obstruction and urethral erosion, the catheter may find its way out of the bladder as it is inserted.

Letting down the bladder

The comments made in relation to urethral catheterization apply equally here. There is no need to decompress the bladder slowly after suprapubic catheterization.

Changing a suprapubic catheter

In many ways, changing a suprapubic catheter is easier than changing a urethral catheter. However, it is very important that the new catheter is ready to be inserted as the old one is removed. A delay of only a few minutes may be enough for the old track to be obliterated as the detrusor fibres contract. As the old catheter is removed, a lubricated catheter of the same size is simply passed down the suprapubic track. The whole length must be passed before inflating the balloon. Should there be a delay following the removal of a suprapubic catheter, and the new one will not pass, then it may be possible to pass a smaller catheter. However, it is usually necessary to dilate the track under a general anaesthetic.

14

Management of Pneumothorax

INTRODUCTION

A pneumothorax is the presence of air or gas in the pleural cavity. This results in partial or total collapse of the lung on that side, depending on the volume of air that enters. Usually, there is a hole in the visceral pleura that allows air to enter the pleural cavity until the pressure gradient across it is equalized. Occasionally, however, a valve-like mechanism exists so that, on inspiration, air enters the pleural cavity but cannot leave on expiration. This results in increasing pressure in the pleural cavity which causes mediastinal shift and compression of the opposite lung. This is a tension pneumothorax and is potentially life threatening. The situation will be discussed further in this chapter.

Pneumothoraces can be divided into two main categories depending on their aetiology: **spontaneous** and **traumatic**. The latter usually occurs after penetrating thoracic injury or a rib fracture and is not specifically discussed in this chapter. In practice, the treatment principles are the same. Spontaneous pneumothorax can be divided into *primary* and *secondary*, depending on whether there is evidence of underlying lung disease as a cause. In a primary spontaneous pneumothorax, there is no evidence of lung disease. Usually, a small bleb on the visceral pleura of the lung ruptures, producing a hole through which air enters the pleural cavity. This is normally a self-limiting air leak. A secondary spontaneous pneumothorax occurs when there is underlying lung disease such as bullous lung disease. In this instance, a bulla rupture causes the air leak. A list of some predisposing factors for the development of a pneumothorax is shown in Box 14.1. Although many pneumothoraces

BOX 14.1   PREDISPOSING FACTORS FOR THE DEVELOPMENT OF A PNEUMOTHORAX

- Thoracic injury
- Emphysema
- Asthma
- Peripheral lung cancer
- Fibrotic lung disease (e.g. fibrosing alveolitis, sarcoidosis or pneumoconioses)
- Active pulmonary tuberculosis
- Connective tissue disorders (e.g. Ehlers–Danlos syndrome or Marfan's syndrome)
- Lung abscess
- Bronchiectasis
- Endometriosis

are self-limiting, occasionally, a bronchopleural fistula develops which gives a persistent air leak.

In 1993, after consultation with over 150 chest physicians and surgeons, the British Thoracic Society drew up guidelines for the management of a spontaneous pneumothorax (Miller and Harvey, 1993). This was as a result of a randomized trial comparing simple aspiration and intercostal tube drainage (Harvey and Prescott, 1994). The guidelines provide a systematic protocol using simple flow diagrams, and the management outlined in this chapter is based on them.

DIAGNOSIS

A diagnosis of pneumothorax should be suspected if a patient presents with sudden onset of unilateral

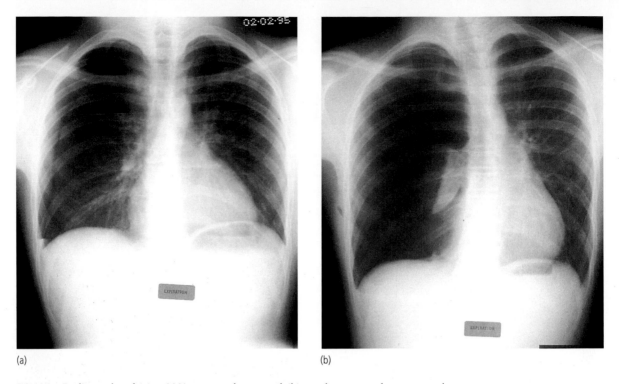

(a)   (b)

FIG 14.1   Radiographs of (a) a 30% pneumothorax and (b) an almost complete pneumothorax.

pleuritic chest pain or increasing breathlessness. It should also be considered as a potential precipitant in patients with an acute exacerbation of their chronic airflow limitation. The features on examination depend on the size of the pneumothorax. Patients with an apical pneumothorax will have little in the way of symptoms. Larger pneumothoraces result in tachypnoea, deviation of the trachea away from the affected side, hyper-resonance, and quiet or absent breath sounds on the affected side. In addition, a tension pneumothorax causes cardiovascular collapse. One should always be alert to this diagnosis if a patient has signs of a pneumothorax associated with hypotension. In this instance, the condition may be life threatening and warrants immediate cannulation of the pneumothorax.

Once the clinical diagnosis of a pneumothorax is suspected, a chest X-ray should be performed to confirm the diagnosis. Both inspiration and expiration films are requested since small apical pneumothoraces will be more evident on an expiratory film. The radiograph should be studied carefully to detect any underlying lung disease and to estimate the size of the pneumothorax. This is expressed as a percentage of the lung collapsed. Figure 14.1(a) shows a radiograph of a 30% pneumothorax and 14.1(b) shows a radiograph of an almost complete pneumothorax.

INITIAL MANAGEMENT

The initial decision to make for a patient with a pneumothorax is whether intervention is needed at all. This is easy if one follows the British Thoracic Society's algorithm (see Fig. 14.2).

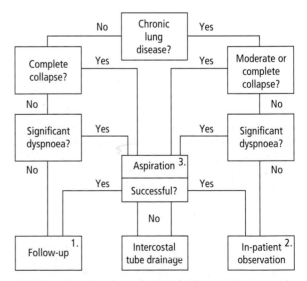

FIG 14.2   Algorithm from the British Thoracic Society guidelines for the management of a pneumothorax.

Algorithm

Notes for annotation of the algorithm

1. A significant proportion of pneumothoraces occur in healthy young people with normal lungs. Providing that there is not total collapse of the lung and the patient is not breathless, no intervention is necessary. The patient can be allowed home but should be told to reattend if they have increasing breathlessness or pleuritic chest pain. They should be reviewed at a thoracic clinic with a follow-up chest X-ray at 2 weeks to ensure re-expansion of the affected lung.

2. Patients with chronic lung disease are more likely to become compromised following a pneumothorax. Therefore, even if they have a pneumothorax not fulfilling the criteria for intervention, they should be observed overnight in hospital and a repeat chest X-ray performed before discharge to ensure that the pneumothorax is not enlarging.

3. In patients who have a pneumothorax which needs intervention, there are two main options: aspiration and intercostal tube drainage. There are advantages and disadvantages for both techniques. Aspirating a pneumothorax is less painful and more cosmetically acceptable for the patient (Archer *et al.*, 1985; Harvey, 1993; Raja and Lalor, 1981). It also is a quicker technique to perform and does not require hospital admission. However, it does not always work and does not solve the problem when a bronchopleural fistula is present, causing a persistent air leak.

In patients with normal lungs who have complete collapse of the lung, an attempt at aspiration of the lung should be made. Partial collapse with symptoms is also an indication for this procedure.

ASPIRATION TECHNIQUE

As with all practical procedures, it is essential to explain fully to the patient what they should expect during the event. Also, it is crucial that the patient is placed in a suitable comfortable position and that the trolley contains all the necessary equipment. An aseptic technique must be used; therefore, an assistant is needed. The items required for the procedure are shown in Box 14.2 (*see also* Fig. 14.3).

Steps

1. The site for the aspiration is chosen. There are two main options regarding this site. The mid-clavicular second intercostal space is normally chosen. However, particularly in women, it can

BOX 14.2 ITEMS REQUIRED FOR ASPIRATION TECHNIQUE

- Small dressing pack
- Antiseptic (e.g. Betadine)
- Sterile towels
- 5–10 mL 1% lignocaine
- 25 G (orange-hubbed) needle
- 16 G (grey) venflon
- 10 mL syringe
- 50 mL Luer-lock syringe
- Three-way tap
- Small plaster
- Sterile surgeon's gloves

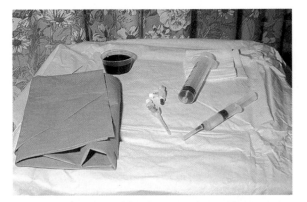

FIG 14.3   Equipment required for the aspiration technique.

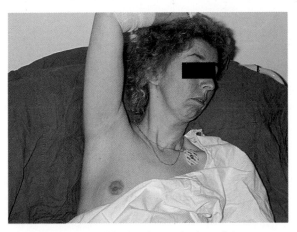

FIG 14.4   Patient positioning for aspiration of the pneumothorax.

be better to use the mid-axillary fourth to sixth intercostal spaces. Occasionally, the pneumothorax may be localized and therefore the site of aspiration will vary.

2. The patient should be positioned lying semi-recumbent with their hand resting behind the head (*see* Fig. 14.4).

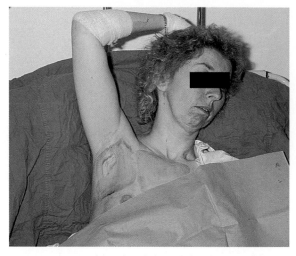

FIG 14.5   Patient cleaned and draped for the procedure.

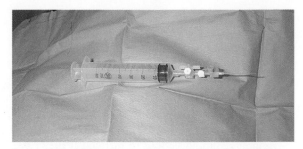

FIG 14.7   Cannula connected to the Luer-lock syringe via the three-way tap.

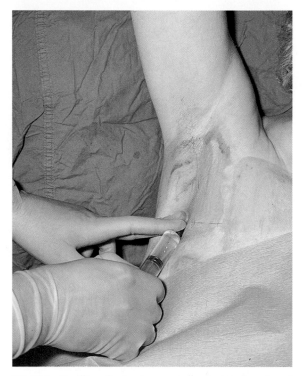

FIG 14.6   Instilling lignocaine to anaesthetize the pleural space. This patient had a localized pneumothorax and therefore the site of aspiration was higher than usual. The photograph also shows air being aspirated, indicating that the lignocaine has been administered right down to the pleural space.

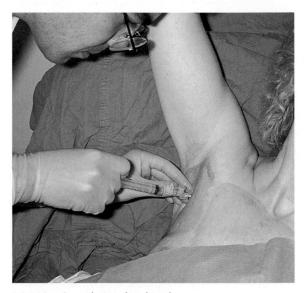

FIG 14.8   Cannulating the pleural space.

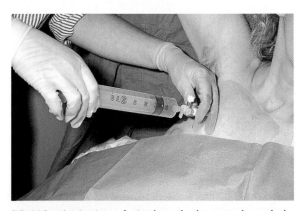

FIG 14.9   Aspiration of air through the cannula and the three-way tap.

3. The chest X-ray should be double-checked to ensure that the correct side is located, and the site for the aspiration of the pneumothorax should then be confirmed by percussion.

4. A check is made to ensure that the patient has no allergy to iodine, and then the whole area is cleaned. Drapes need to be placed around the sterile field (see Fig. 14.5).

5. The area is anaesthetized. Using a 25 G needle, an intradermal bleb of local anaesthetic is raised. The subcutaneous tissues should then be infiltrated down to the pleura using 5–10 mL of 1%

lignocaine. It is important to remember that the neurovascular bundle runs beneath each rib and that the syringe should be aspirated before injection of the anaesthetic (*see* Fig. 14.6).

6. By maintaining gentle suction on the syringe, it is easy to recognize when the pleural cavity has been entered since bubbles of air will be aspirated. The needle and syringe can then be removed.

7. Connection of the cannula. The three-way tap is attached to the Luer-lock syringe and placed close to hand (*see* Fig. 14.7). Using a 16 French-gauge cannula attached to a 5 mL syringe, the pleural space is re-entered (*see* Fig. 14.8). Once air is freely aspirated, the needle is removed from the cannula and the syringe. The thumb is placed over the cannula to prevent more air entering the pleural space. The plastic cannula is connected to the three-way tap and the 50 mL Luer-lock syringe system (already set up). By applying suction, a syringeful of air can be aspirated which then can be voided into the atmosphere using the other port of the three-way tap, without disconnecting the syringe (*see* Fig. 14.9).

8. Air should be removed until resistance is felt or when 2500 mL has been aspirated. It is important to reassure the patient that they may experience coughing or pleuritic chest pain as the lung inflates. If resistance is felt when only a small amount of air has been removed, then the cannula should be withdrawn and replaced since it probably has become kinked.

9. The chest X-ray is repeated following the procedure in order to confirm that the pneumothorax has resolved.

10. Many patients can be discharged but, occasionally, depending on the patient's social situation and tolerance of the procedure, they may need to be admitted overnight. Follow-up should be arranged at a chest clinic in 2 weeks time.

If the aspiration technique fails, then the insertion of an intercostal drain is required.

INTERCOSTAL TUBE DRAINAGE TECHNIQUE

Again, it is imperative to explain to the patient what is happening, both prior to and during the procedure. To ensure adequate pain relief, premedication with intramuscular pethidine is useful. In exceptional circumstances, for example particularly anxious patients, the use of a short-acting sedative (e.g. midazolam) can be of benefit. However, we do not advocate the routine use of sedation since this may cause respiratory embarrassment, and also requires the help of another assistant, who is experienced in sedation, to observe the patient.

BOX 14.3   ITEMS REQUIRED FOR INTERCOSTAL TUBE DRAINAGE

- Sterile pack for intercostal tube drainage
- 24 G intercostal drain
- Intercostal drain connection tubing
- Glass bottle
- 200 mL sterile water
- Sterile towels
- Sterile surgeon's gloves
- Antiseptic (e.g. Betadine)
- Surgical blade
- Sterile blunt-ended forceps, stitch holder and scissors
- 10–15 mL 1% lignocaine
- 25 G (orange-hubbed) needle
- 21 G (green-hubbed) needle
- 20 mL syringe
- Suture (e.g. 1/0 silk)
- Adhesive tap
- Sterile gauze

Steps

1. The trolley should be checked to make certain that all the equipment listed in Box 14.3 is available. The glass bottle has to be filled with sterile water to the indicated level in order to form the underwater seal. All the tube connections should be checked to ensure that they are a good fit in order to prevent an air leak.

2. The skin is prepared and draped as described for the aspiration technique.

3. The position of the site of the chest drain should be in the mid-axillary line in the fourth to sixth intercostal space.

4. Local anaesthetic should be administered and the incision is made as described in Chapter 15 for insertion of a chest drain. It should be large enough to allow a finger to enter the wound but less than 2 cm long. A large incision means that the drain does not fit snugly in the hole and an air leak can result.

5. For a patient with a pneumothorax, a 20–24 French-gauge tube should be used. Ideally, the tube should lie in the apex of the lung. Therefore, the tube is inserted with the trocar *in situ* along the fashioned tract (*see* Chapter 15 for details regarding the blunt dissection). Once the tube enters the pleural cavity, it is aimed upwards and advanced slowly. The tube should be slid off the trocar until resistance is felt and it cannot be advanced further. At that stage, the tube is pulled back about 1 cm; this ensures that it is not right up against the mediastinum or chest wall. The tube is clamped while the trocar is removed to prevent air entering the pleural cavity.

6. The drain should then be connected to the under-water seal and the clamp removed.
7. The drain is checked to ensure that it is bubbling and that it swings with respiration. Again, the patient should be reassured that they may experience chest tightness or pain as the lung inflates.
8. The drain should be sutured in place as described in Chapter 15. The securing of the chest drain is crucial: it should be taped at the site of entry and a loop of tube should be taped to the patient's abdomen. If, for any reason, the tube is pulled, the pressure will then be transmitted only as far as the abdomen.
9. Adequate analgesia should be prescribed.
10. A chest X-ray is repeated to ensure that the tube is in a suitable position in the apex of the lung and that the lung has re-expanded.

Management of the chest drain

The drainage bottle must be kept below the level of the tube in the patient's chest at all times. The chest drain needs to be *in situ* until the lung is fully expanded. This can be checked by asking the patient to cough while observing the underwater seal. If there is bubbling, then the pneumothorax has not resolved. Once bubbling has ceased for 24 h, a chest X-ray is repeated to ensure that the lung is expanded radiologically, and then the drain is removed.

The chest drain should not be clamped unless the bottle breaks. This means that the drain does not need to be clamped when the patient is transported, for example to the X-ray department. This is because if the lung is re-expanded, it will go down again if the tube is clamped whilst there is a persistent air leak into the pleural cavity. Also, if the patient has a bronchopleural fistula and the chest drain is clamped, this could potentially precipitate a tension pneumothorax.

Removal of the chest drain

To remove the chest drain, an aseptic technique should be used. Lignocaine (2 mL, 1%) is infiltrated around the tube and a suture placed across the incision. The patient is requested to hold their breath in inspiration and then the drain is removed while tightening the suture over the entry site. A chest X-ray should then be performed to ensure that the lung has remained inflated. The patient may then be discharged with an out-patient appointment made for 2 weeks later. It is important to instruct the patient to return if either they become acutely short of breath, or develop pleuritic chest pain. The patient must also be told not to travel in a pressurized aircraft until they have been discharged from the chest clinic. This is because the trapped air in the

---

BOX 14.4 CAUSES OF TUBE DRAINAGE FAILURE

- Drain too small
- Inadequate suction
- Persistent air leak
- Inappropriate clamping of the drain
- Removal of the drain too early (i.e. when still bubbling)
- Bronchial obstruction (e.g. mucus plug or tumour) preventing lung expansion

---

pleural cavity will expand if the patient is in an aircraft pressurized at lower than atmospheric pressure. This would then cause worsening of the pneumothorax.

Problems with chest drains

There are a variety of reasons why tube drainage may fail. Box 14.4 lists the most common problems.

The following guidelines suggest how to interpret different problems with chest drains and how to rectify them.

Fluid level not swinging

This occurs if the tube is not patent. The possible causes are:

1. the lung is fully expanded;
2. the drain is blocked;
3. the drain is in an inadequate position.

In this situation, a plan should be made to perform a chest X-ray. If this confirms that the lung is expanded, then the tube is removed. If the lung is not expanded, and the drain appears to be up against the mediastinum or chest wall, the tube is withdrawn slightly. The drain should never be advanced further into the chest as this could introduce infection. If there is any doubt at all, the drain should be removed and replaced using a different incision site.

Drain continues to bubble

This means that the pneumothorax has not resolved. Therefore, the chest X-ray must be repeated. If the pneumothorax is improving, the patient is then reassessed the following day. If the pneumothorax is unchanged, then the chest drain must be placed on suction using a low-pressure/high-volume pump (e.g. a Vernon Thompson pump) with the pressure set at 15–20 cmH$_2$O.

If there is still bubbling of air while the chest drain is on suction, this means that there is a persistent air leak. Causes of this include:

1. a bronchopleural fistula;
2. a hole in the tube outside the chest wall;
3. the incision in the chest wall is too lax;
4. a leak in the system.

A bronchopleural fistula occurs when there is a communication between the airways and the pleural cavity. To establish the cause of the air leak, confirmation that the chest drain remains in a good position is made by performing a chest X-ray. The entry hole is checked to ensure that it is not too lax and, if it is, another suture is placed across the entry site. All the connections are checked for tightness of fit. If both the site and entry hole of the drain seem correct, then the drain is kept on suction and the patient is referred to a respiratory physician.

If a bronchopleural fistula has developed, then a pleurodesis may solve the problem. There are two main techniques: medical and surgical. The medical technique involves the administration of a sclerosant down the chest drain. The sclerosant is an irritant, such as tetracycline, and causes fibrous adhesions to form between the visceral and parietal pleura. These then obliterate the pleural space and stick the visceral pleura to the chest wall. This method may be employed if there is a persistent air leak but the lung is seen to be expanded on the chest X-ray. If, however, there is a continuing air leak and a persistent pneumothorax despite the lung being on adequate suction, a surgical thoroscopic procedure will be needed. In young patients with repeated unilateral pneumothoraces, one should proceed directly to a definitive surgical procedure.

Surgical emphysema

Surgical emphysema is the presence of air in the subcutaneous tissues and can be alarming to both the doctor and the patient. It usually occurs because the entry hole through the pleura is too large. Fortunately, it is an uncommon complication and the simple measure of placing the drain on suction usually rectifies the situation. If it does not, then referral to a respiratory physician should be made. Very rarely, there may be so much surgical emphysema that it causes respiratory embarrassment which is recognized by stridor and dyspnoea. In this situation, emergency decompression is indicated. This is achieved by placing small subcutaneous incisions below the clavicles and milking the air out through these incisions.

Haemothorax

A small amount of blood-stained fluid may accumulate in the chest drain tube. However, in the event of rapid bleeding filling the tube, emergency measures must be undertaken. The bleeding may be due to damage to an intercostal blood vessel on insertion of the drain, or contusion of the lung itself. The patient must be adequately resuscitated and urgent help obtained from a thoracic surgeon.

CONCLUSIONS

This management plan provides straightforward instructions for the successful management of a pneumothorax for both the patient and doctor alike. Box 14.5 indicates situations where a specialist respiratory opinion should be sought. The aspiration technique will treat many types of pneumothorax. Intercostal tube drainage is needed if the aspiration technique fails or there is evidence of a bronchopleural fistula. Surgical referral is still needed for some of the more complicated pneumothoraces with a persistent air leak. A respiratory referral should be made for patients who have repeated pneumothoraces.

BOX 14.5   SITUATIONS WHEN A RESPIRATORY OPINION SHOULD BE SOUGHT

- Any problem with tube insertion
- Haemothorax
- Tube still bubbling at 24–48 h
- Tube not bubbling and lung not expanded
- Subcutaneous emphysema
- Bilateral pneumothorax, tension pneumothorax or a second pneumothorax

REFERENCES

Archer, G.J., Hamilton, A.A.D., Upadhyay, M., Finlay, M. and Grace, P.M. 1985: Results of simple aspiration of pneumothoraces. *British Journal of Diseases of the Chest* 79, 177–82.

Harvey, J.E. 1993: Comparison of simple aspiration with intercostal drainage in the management of spontaneous pneumothorax. *Thorax* 48, 430–1.

Harvey, J. and Prescott, R.J. 1994: Simple aspiration versus intercostal tube drainage for spontaneous pneumothorax in patients with normal lungs. *British Medical Journal* 309, 1338–9.

Miller, A.C. and Harvey, J.E. 1993: Guidelines for the management of spontaneous pneumothorax. *British Medical Journal* 307, 114–16.

Raja, O.G. and Lalor, A.J. 1981: Simple aspiration of spontaneous pneumothorax. *British Journal of Diseases of the Chest* 75, 207–8.

15

Pleural Aspiration and Biopsy

INTRODUCTION

The techniques of aspiration of a pleural effusion and biopsy of the parietal pleura are important diagnostic skills that can usefully and rewardingly be acquired, under supervision, by most medical house staff on busy medical or respiratory teams. Aspiration of large volumes of pleural fluid may be necessary as an urgent therapeutic procedure for the relief of breathlessness. The technique is identical in principle to that for aspirating air from pneumothoraces (*see* Chapter 14).

INDICATIONS

Pleural fluid may accumulate as the result of many local or systemic diseases. In a few cases, the cause may be apparent: for example recurrent pleural effusions associated with repeated occurrence of congestive heart failure. However, even in such a situation, the demonstration of a transudate would be reassuring and would prompt an increase in antifailure medication, but an aspiration yielding blood-stained fluid suggestive of pulmonary infarction has additional therapeutic implications.

Unfortunately, even after a full (including occupational) history with a thorough physical examination and a chest radiograph, the cause of the effusion often remains elusive and further evaluation is necessary. First, diagnostic aspiration of some fluid should be performed together with biopsy of the parietal pleura. In moderate or large effusions this should pose no difficulty, but small loculated or subpulmonary effusions may require localization by ultrasound scanning and these are outside the scope of this chapter, although the basic principles remain the same.

PLEURAL ASPIRATION

Pleural aspiration is a simple procedure involving the use of little more equipment than is required for venepuncture (Fig. 15.1). It is well tolerated, relatively safe and can be performed in an out-patient clinic. The technique is diagnostically important because it usually enables pleural effusions to be categorized as one of two fundamentally different pathophysiological states: inflammatory exudate or passive transudate.

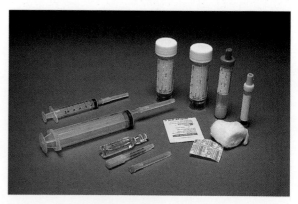

FIG 15.1   Equipment required for simple diagnostic aspiration of a pleural effusion.

TECHNIQUE

The patient should be fully informed and reassured at every stage of the procedure. With appropriate regard for warmth and modesty, the patient is seated and positioned with the trunk square and the arms supported on a table or over the back of a chair padded with pillows (Fig. 15.2). The approach should be posterior and should be made in an intercostal space below the level of dullness to percussion, about 10 cm lateral to the midline. It is important that the approach is above the body of the rib, rather than below, because of the site of the neurovascular bundle (Fig. 15.3). This should be determined by palpation; it may be helpful to mark this site with a skin-marker pen.

The skin is cleaned with spirit and 1% lignocaine is introduced into the skin with an orange-hubbed 25 G needle. A larger blue-hubbed 20 G needle is used to anaesthetize the intercostal tissue down to and including the pleura. Aspiration of some pleural fluid when completing the local anaesthetic injection is a reassuring indication that the site has been correctly chosen.

A green-hubbed 21 G needle attached to a 30 mL syringe is used for the diagnostic aspiration. It is inserted perpendicular to the skin and passed through the anaesthetized tissue (Fig. 15.4). A loss of resistance to penetration of the needle or 'give' is felt as the needle enters the pleural space. Aspiration of sufficient fluid to fill the syringe is adequate for all initial diagnostic tests to be performed and the

technique should be sufficiently atraumatic that an effusion is not stained with blood. On completion of aspiration, a small plaster is used as the only dressing required.

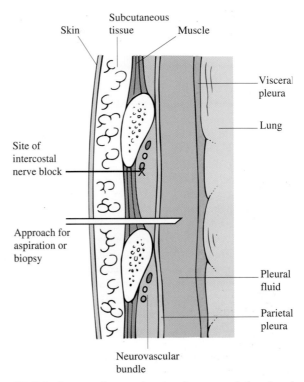

FIG 15.3 Intercostal space showing the approach for pleural aspiration, biopsy and intercostal nerve blocks in relation to the intercostal neurovascular bundle and the body of the ribs.

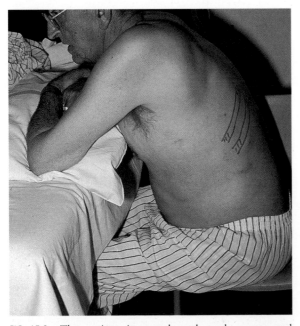

FIG 15.2 The patient is seated, and made warm and comfortable. Aspiration can now proceed at the marked site.

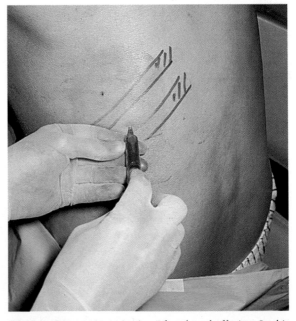

FIG 15.4 Diagnostic aspiration of a pleural effusion. In this case, the fluid is bloodstained because of the underlying pathology.

If no fluid is aspirated, a further attempt should be made in a lower intercostal space (Box 15.1). If there is still no yield of fluid, an approach along the anaesthetized track should be made, using the largest-gauge venepuncture needle available, in case an unsuspected viscid empyema is present. If these attempts are unsuccessful, the case should be discussed with radiologists because further investigations (particularly ultrasound imaging) are helpful in establishing the presence and location of pleural fluid. On scanning the patient, the radiologist can at least mark the skin at a site overlying the maximum depth of collected fluid, if not assist a further attempt at aspiration by real-time scanning. Care should, of course, be taken that the position of the patient for a subsequent aspiration attempt is identical to that when the ultrasound imaging was performed. A persistent 'dry tap' in the presence of fluid apparent on a plain chest radiograph is highly suggestive of an empyema which has typical ultrasonic appearances.

Aspiration of volumes exceeding 50 mL is rarely required for diagnosis but volumes up to 1 L can be removed in one sitting for symptomatic relief of breathlessness. Drainage of such large volumes is relatively time consuming but can be achieved in one of two ways. The use of plastic cannulae, rather than metal needles, is desirable, in case the patient moves or coughs unexpectedly.

The *first technique uses a normal intravenous cannula*, introduced as in intravenous cannulation, under local anaesthesia. A three-way tap, connected to a large syringe and a length of sterile tubing (such as a truncated giving set) is then attached (Fig. 15.5). Fluid can then be aspirated from the chest and expelled via the tubing into a suitable receptacle. Aspiration should be stopped if the patient experiences discomfort, if resistance to aspiration is felt by the operator or when 1 L of fluid has been collected. The only problem with plastic cannulae is that they tend to bend and care is required in supporting the cannulae during aspirations. This technique is identical with that for aspirating pneumothoraces.

Alternatively, with local anaesthesia, a pigtailed suprapubic or other similar catheter can be introduced aseptically, and then connected up to a suitable drainage bag. Drainage can then be achieved by a siphon effect with the rate controlled by a clamp.

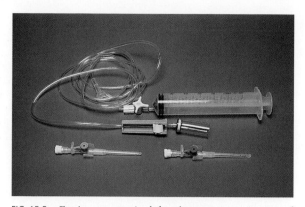

FIG 15.5   Equipment required for therapeutic aspiration of large volumes of pleural fluid. The use of a plastic cannula, rather than a metal needle, is desirable because the procedure is relatively lengthy and the patient may move or cough unexpectedly There are now commercially available prepackaged kits with a similar range of equipment.

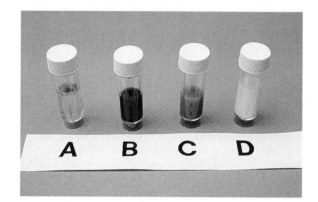

FIG 15.6   Appearances of pleural fluid: (A) serous, straw coloured; (B) bloodstained; (C) purulent; (D) chylous (*see also* Table 15.1).

TABLE 15.1   The gross appearance of aspirated pleural fluid may suggest the diagnosis

APPEARANCE OF FLUID	CONDITION INDICATED

Serous, straw coloured	Transudate
	Exudate:
	    infection (including tuberculosis),
	    neoplasia,
	    pulmonary embolism,
	    connective tissue disorder

Bloodstained	Pulmonary infarction Malignancy Trauma
Purulent	Empyema

Chylous	Lymphatic obstruction:
	    carcinoma
	    lymphoma

TABLE 15.2   Principal tests for the investigation of aspirated fluid

	TEST[a]	COMMENT
Biochemistry	Total protein*	<30 g/L: transudate; >30 g/L: exudate
		Best related to blood protein level (exudate if protein >50% total blood protein)
	Lactate dehydrogenase	Occasionally helpful in addition to the above
	Glucose*	Low in rheumatoid or parapneumonic effusions, sometimes malignancy
	Amylase*	Higher than in blood following pancreatitis and remaining elevated even after blood levels have normalized. Consider pancreatitis, particularly in left-sided effusions even if no history of abdominal pain.
		Elevated in pancreatic cysts, oesophageal rupture or malignancy
	pH	Rarely used
	Differential cell count*	Helpful
Cytology	Malignant cells ?*	May be difficult to differentiate reactive mesothelial cells from some malignant cells. Liaise with cytologist as special staining techniques marker studies or electron microscopy may help
Microbiology	Gram stain*	Quick, simple and helpful
	Culture*	Both aerobic and anaerobic. Consider fungal aetiology
	Bacterial antigens*	Usually tested for pneumococcal antigen. Not available at all centres
	Stain and culture for mycobacteria*	Poor yield – much better to obtain pleural biopsy for histology and culture
Immunology	Rheumatoid factor	Not specific for rheumatoid diseases
	Complement levels	Not specific for connective tissue disorders as low levels also found in malignancy and infection
	Tumour-associated antigens	Not specific for malignancy

[a]This list is not exhaustive – the most clinically helpful tests are marked by an asterisk and should be considered as routine on all pleural fluid specimens.

Aspirated fluid: appearance and investigation

The gross appearance of the fluid may suggest possible causes (Fig. 15.6, Table 15.1). The most useful investigations that can be performed are outlined in Table 15.2. The most important are those used in differentiating a transudate from an exudate. The distinction can often be made from the protein concentration alone or by relating fluid protein concentration to levels of protein in peripheral whole blood; similar comparison of blood lactate dehydrogenase (LDH) activity confers little additional bonus. Such demarcation in transudate/exudate based on protein concentration is not always complete. Where differentiation is possible, this is diagnostically important. A transudate shifts the focus of attention from the pleura to a multisystem disorder, whereas an exudate implies local and often serious pathology. In the latter case, more invasive investigation is frequently required, commencing with a pleural biopsy in order to obtain pleural tissue for histological and microbiological examination.

PLEURAL BIOPSY

The standard pleural biopsy is performed percutaneously using an Abram's biopsy needle (Fig. 15.7), but only if pleural fluid is present. Pleural biopsy should always be considered when the decision to perform a pleural fluid aspiration is made. Both percutaneous 'Trucut' needle biopsy of the pleura and thoracoscopic pleural biopsy are techniques for experienced operators and are not considered further here.

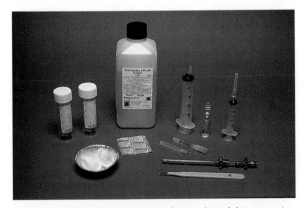

FIG 15.7   Additional equipment for a pleural biopsy using an Abram's needle as described (see text).

TECHNIQUE

This procedure is more invasive than simple aspiration alone. The patient should be placed in a similar position to that for pleural aspiration (see above) and a posterior approach should be adopted, providing that the effusion is not loculated elsewhere.

The skin is prepared as for pleural aspiration but a larger area should be cleaned. Lignocaine (1%) is liberally used to anaesthetize the skin and the pleura. If anaesthesia is inadequate, the biopsy will be uncomfortable and distressing. Total anaesthesia of all the pleura likely to be biopsied is perhaps an unrealistic goal but the careful placement of two intercostal nerve blocks helps to achieve adequate anaesthesia. This involves placing 1 mL of lignocaine, with a narrow-gauge needle, just inferior and deep to the lower border of the ribs bordering the selected intercostal space.

At this point, and while allowing time for the anaesthetic to act, the biopsy equipment (needle, tap and syringe) should be assembled and the operator should ensure that he/she is comfortable handling the apparatus (practice is useful) and that the system is working smoothly. The following checks, in particular, should be made:

■ The reference knob on the hexagonal outer guard should be in line with the biopsy needle.
■ The cutting action of the inner tube must be smooth.

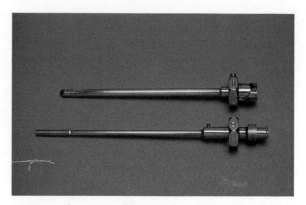

FIG 15.8 Abram's needle. Note the outer (top) and inner (bottom) tubes, the biopsy window and the reference knob on the hexagonal guard of the outer tube.

■ When screwed home, the inner tube should cut and close the window of the outer tube.
■ When screwed back, this window should open to allow aspiration of fluid, intrusion of pleura or extraction of the biopsy after it has been performed (Fig. 15.8).

Once anaesthesia is achieved, a stab incision is made with a sterile pointed scalpel blade, perpendicular to the skin and just above the upper border of a rib (Fig. 15.9). The incision is then deepened by blunt dissection with either fingers or artery forceps as needed. In due course, and with the window closed and the inner tube positioned well home, the Abram's biopsy

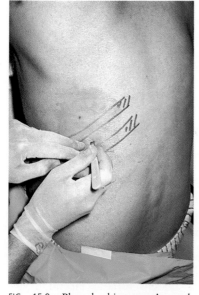

FIG 15.9 Pleural biopsy. A stab incision is made into anaesthetized skin before introduction of Abram's needle assembly. The needle assembly is not sharp enough to be used to make a track.

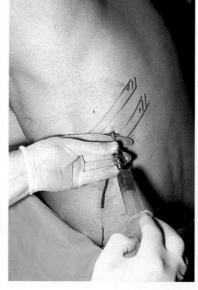

FIG 15.10 Abram's needle introduced into the chest; aspiration of fluid confirms the position.

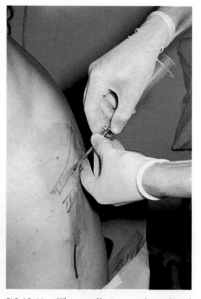

FIG 15.11 The needle is steeply inclined just before the assembly is dragged back along the parietal pleura for the biopsy. The needle was inserted immediately over a rib, but the traction on the skin gives the appearance of insertion under a rib.

needle is introduced with gentle pressure, gently popping through the pleura into the effusion. Correct positioning of the needle can be established by opening the window and aspirating pleural fluid (Fig. 15.10). The biopsy needle should not be pushed too hard; it is not sharp enough to make a track of its own.

The needle and syringe should now be steeply inclined (almost vertically) with the needle caudal, the window against the parietal pleura, the syringe uppermost and the reference knob directed away from the patient (Fig. 15.11). The lip of the window is then dragged cranially along the chest wall until the gentle resistance of the pleura is felt, at which point the window is closed, thereby trapping a fold of pleura. The needle is removed and the incision is covered with gauze.

A small needle is normally used to extract the biopsy from the open window and the biopsy is placed in fixative for histological examination. Normal pleura has a silver-grey sheen (Fig. 15.12). Thickened pleural tissue offers more resistance to biopsy than does normal tissue. If muscle fibres are repeatedly obtained, the inclination of the needle is insufficiently steep.

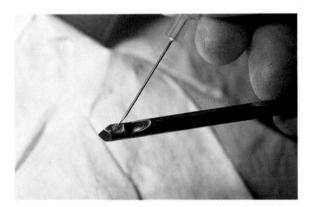

FIG 15.12   Silver-grey appearance of a fresh pleural biopsy.

This biopsy procedure should be repeated with the needle directed down and to the left, and down and to the right, in order to yield a further two samples. It is important never to biopsy above the level of approach. One biopsy sample for microbiological (especially mycobacterial) culture should be placed in a sterile universal container with a drop of normal saline (to prevent drying) and should be transported swiftly to the laboratory.

Most biopsies are performed in order to provide parietal pleura for histological examination when malignancy is suspected. Pleural biopsy with histological examination and culture is even more useful when tuberculosis is suspected, and it is good practice always to obtain an extra biopsy for mycobacterial culture.

BOX 15.2   COMPLICATIONS OF PLEURAL BIOPSY

- Vasovagal attack
- Bleeding
- Pneumothorax
- Collapse (due to any of the above or re-expansion pulmonary oedema)

COMPLICATIONS

Bleeding is rarely a problem if aspiration and biopsy are avoided in patients with a clotting disorder (international normalized ratio should be less than 1.3 and the platelet count should exceed $60 \times 10^9/L$). Accidental biopsy of the intercostal vessels should be avoided by choosing the line of insertion above a rib, taking care with blunt dissection and by obtaining biopsies with a needle directed inferior to the point of insertion.

Pneumothorax is the commonest complication, although intervention is rarely indicated. Laceration of the visceral pleura should be avoided by not draining an effusion completely using a metal needle. Moreover, complete drainage of an effusion also precludes subsequent repeat pleural biopsy.

'*Collapse*' of the patient may be caused by pneumothorax, haemothorax or re-expansion pulmonary oedema. The latter is avoided simply by never removing more than 1 L of aspirate at a single sitting. Occasionally, a vasovagal reaction occurs as a needle passes through the pleura; this is rare and unavoidable but can take the operator by surprise.

NON-DIAGNOSTIC PLEURAL BIOPSY

This is an indication for seeking specialist help. Clearly, if none of the samples contain pleura then there is a problem with technique, usually that of insufficient inclination of the Abram's biopsy needle. If the histopathologists describe the pleural biopsy as showing chronic inflammation, then liaison with them is necessary regarding whether a further sample or additional staining techniques are necessary (could it be mesothelioma?). In this situation, or in the case of a histologically unremarkable pleural biopsy in the presence of a serous exudative pleural effusion, the question of whether to repeat blind Abram's biopsy or biopsy under direct vision via thoracoscopy will need to be discussed with the local respiratory medical or surgical service.

EMPYEMA

This is a particular, though fortunately relatively uncommon, type of pleural effusion that poses a number of problems. First of all, it is uncommon and the diagnosis may not be considered even when on the plain chest radiograph there is the typical D-shaped pleural-based shadow. In this situation, there should be prompt confirmation of the presence of purulent fluid. Blind aspiration, even with a large-bore metal needle, may be difficult because of the viscid nature of the pleural contents. The early involvement of the ultrasound service should be elicited as the typical appearances of loculated debris-rich pleural fluid will be apparent, and also the best site for aspiration can be indicated. The respiratory medicine team should be involved at an early stage as drainage may be necessary by repeated aspiration or by the insertion of a wide-bore intercostal drain with intra-pleural fibinolysis.

16

Joint Aspiration

INTRODUCTION

Joint aspiration is a simple and invaluable procedure for the diagnosis and treatment of joint disease. It is particularly required for diagnosis and management of the acute 'hot, red joint' – a medical emergency. The knee is the commonest site to require aspiration, although any non-axial joint is readily accessible. The technique involves only a basic knowledge of anatomy and should not be unduly painful for the patient. Provided sterile equipment and a sensible, aseptic approach are used, it is a safe procedure that can be readily undertaken by junior medical staff.

INDICATIONS

Principal indications for joint aspiration are listed in Box 16.1. An important requirement is the **diagnosis of acute synovitis**. It is only by examination of synovial fluid (SF) that joint sepsis or crystal-associated synovitis (gout or 'pseudogout') can be accurately diagnosed. This particularly relates to presentation with acute monoarthritis (one joint). However, it is also relevant for acute oligoarthritis (two to four joints), or for the patient with pre-existing chronic polyarthritis, such as rheumatoid disease, who develops a 'flare' of synovitis limited to only one or a few joints. In all these situations, sepsis requires urgent consideration. Important clinical features ('red flags') that always require consideration of sepsis include:

- any *acute synovitis* in one or a few joints, but especially in *patients at increased risk* of joint sepsis, for example patients with rheumatoid arthritis, diabetes, or compromised immunity due to disease or drugs (in adults, sepsis most commonly occurs in joints with pre-existing damage);

BOX 16.1   INDICATIONS FOR JOINT ASPIRATION

Diagnosis
Acute synovitis
- Sepsis
- Crystals
  — common:
     monosodium urate (gout)
     calcium pyrophosphate ('pseudogout')
  — rare:
     other crystals (e.g. oxalate or cholesterol)
- Haemorrhage

Chronic arthropathy
- Crystals (monosodium urate or calcium pyrophosphate)

Treatment
Common
- Reduce intra-articular pressure
- Injection of steroid

Less common (mainly by rheumatologists)
- Recurrent aspiration for sepsis
- Saline lavage for resistant arthropathy

- rapidly *progressive symptoms* in a single joint;
- *additive joint involvement* (e.g. first metatarsophalangeal joint, followed by ankle and then knee involvement on the same side);
- synovitis with *overlying erythema* – a sign of periarticular inflammation that particularly accompanies sepsis or crystals.

Combined symptoms and signs of synovitis include marked early-morning and inactivity stiffness, increased warmth, soft-tissue swelling, effusion, joint-line tenderness and pain, and restriction in a 'stress' pattern (i.e. progressively worse towards the extremes of the range of movement). Haemarthrosis due to a bleeding disorder often results in an acute, tense effusion with marked stress pain and restriction, but little increased warmth and no associated erythema. Aspiration of chronically inflamed joints, or even asymptomatic joints during intercritical periods, may be undertaken as a non-urgent procedure for diagnosis of gout.

Frequent aspiration, two or three times daily, may be required as part of the management of septic arthritis. However, surgical drainage should be undertaken early (within 36 h) if rapid reaccumulation or loculation resistant to simple aspiration occurs. This and the other less-common listed indications are best undertaken by specialist teams. A prosthetic joint should not be aspirated without prior consultation with an orthopaedic surgeon or rheumatologist. Similarly, aspiration of joints in children should only be undertaken by experienced personnel.

Aspiration of SF from a tensely swollen joint, due to synovitis or haemarthrosis, may quickly relieve severe pain by reducing intra-articular hypertension. However, rapid reaccumulation of SF or blood may be problematic. If the patient is known to have a haemorrhagic disorder (e.g. haemophilia), the bleeding tendency should be corrected *prior* to aspiration to reduce the chance of rebleeding. In the situation of aggressive synovitis (e.g. crystal-associated synovitis, reactive arthritis or rheumatoid arthritis), reaccumulation of SF may be temporarily reduced by combining aspiration with an intra-articular injection of long-acting steroid. However, this should only be done when the diagnosis is clear, often as a second procedure following the exclusion of sepsis.

GENERAL PROCEDURE

An aseptic technique is mandatory (Box 16.2). The crucial aspects of this are the use of sterile equipment and clean hands. Gloves should be worn to protect

BOX 16.2 GENERAL PRINCIPLES OF JOINT ASPIRATION

- Explain procedure to patient
- Position patient appropriately (supported, relaxed)
- Use aseptic technique
  — wash hands
  — clean skin with alcohol swab
- Needle size
  — large joint: 21 (or 19) G
  — small joint: 23 (or 25) G
- Avoid surface blood vessels
- Do not aspirate through potentially infected skin/cellulitis

the operator in high-risk situations (e.g. possible risk of HIV or hepatitis) and some would advocate their routine use. However, there is no need to gown up or go to theatre — it is perfectly acceptable to carry out the procedure on the general ward or in the clinic.

The rationale and nature of the procedure should be explained to the patient. A clear indication of the expected level of discomfort and the symptom relief that may follow should be included. The more informed and relaxed the patient is, the less of a 'procedure' it becomes. Although aspiration involves a needle-prick and some discomfort, in general it should be no more painful than venepuncture. This is especially true for large joints, such as the knee, ankle or glenohumeral joint, and joints with moderate to large effusions. The procedure itself is relatively quick and any discomfort should be short lived. Although florid acute gout often associates with extreme tenderness, relief from aspiration is immediate, dramatic and inevitably appreciated. The patient is positioned on a couch or chair with the region of interest supported sufficiently that the muscles can comfortably relax. The surface anatomy and joint landmarks are identified and the site and angle of entry are confirmed. Obvious surface blood vessels and varicose veins should be avoided. A joint must not be aspirated via cellulitic skin as this increases the risk of infecting the joint. The skin site is cleaned with an alcohol swab and dabbed dry with a sterile cotton wool ball (to prevent uncomfortable stinging when the skin is punctured). Local anaesthetic (spray, cream or injection) is not usually administered for adults.

Large joints, such as the knee and shoulder, can be aspirated using a 21 G green-hubbed needle although a larger needle may be required to readily aspirate very purulent SF. A 23 G blue-hubbed or 25 G orange-hubbed needle is appropriate for smaller joints. The size of the syringe will be determined by the estimate of the volume to be aspirated. In general, smaller syringes (5, 10 or 20 mL) are easiest to operate. The plunger of large syringes (30 or 50 mL) may prove difficult to withdraw, and Luer (screw) locks may cause problems of air entry or difficult disengagement for subsequent steroid injection. For large effusions, it is often easier to disengage, empty and reuse a 20 mL syringe than to employ a larger barrel size. If aspiration and steroid injection are being combined, the steroid is drawn into a second (usually 1 or 2 mL) syringe just prior to aspiration and kept close to hand, capped with a sheathed needle.

The patient should be warned to expect the needle-prick and, without undue delay, the needle is inserted through the skin in the desired direction. The patient may experience some discomfort as the needle pierces the skin and joint capsule. Marked discomfort usually reflects inaccurate placement, for example direct contact with periosteum. A slight 'give' is usually felt as the needle enters the joint cavity. Very little resistance should be encountered – difficulty advancing the needle suggests that it is in the wrong position. If there is marked resistance or discomfort, the needle should be withdrawn slightly, the landmarks reassessed, the syringe and needle redirected and another attempt made to advance gently. When it is felt that the needle is correctly positioned, the plunger should be withdrawn, being very careful not to dislodge the needle. Aspiration of SF confirms correct placement.

In most situations, as much SF as possible should be removed. If the flow of SF becomes intermittent or stops, this may be due to:

■ temporary obstruction by synovial fronds;
■ blockage by fibrin and debris;
■ loculation of SF;
■ displacement of the needle outside the joint cavity.

If this happens, a very small amount of SF should simply be injected back from the barrel of the syringe. This often clears the needle of debris or overlying fronds, permitting the aspiration to continue unimpeded. If this manoeuvre is unsuccessful, the needle should be withdrawn slightly and then reinserted to see if this clears the problem. If there is very troublesome blockage of the needle (e.g. with fibrinous 'rice bodies'; Fig. 16.1) that is greatly delaying the procedure, it may be necessary to withdraw altogether and try again with a larger-bore needle.

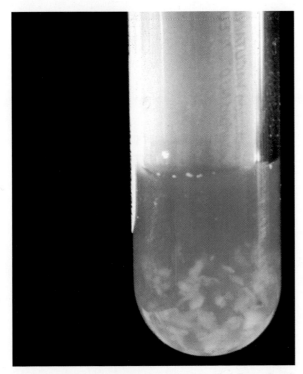

FIG 16.1 Fibrinous 'rice bodies' in bloodstained SF aspirated from the knee of a patient with long-standing rheumatoid arthritis.

If concomitant steroid injection is required, it is often an advantage not to aspirate to dryness. Leaving a little SF behind keeps the 'joint space' open and reduces the risk of needle displacement. At the end of aspiration, the end of the needle is held firmly with one hand and the barrel of the syringe disengaged with the other; then, the syringe with the predrawn steroid is attached. Great care should be taken not to dislodge the needle during this changeover. The steroid can now be injected. Correct placement is suggested by:

■ ability to aspirate SF again;
■ low resistance to injection.

If there is resistance to injection, the needle should be withdrawn slightly, the landmarks redefined and the needle reinserted in the correct direction.

At the end of aspiration or injection, the needle is withdrawn and pressure applied firmly over the puncture site with a cotton wool ball until local skin bleeding has stopped. A plaster is optional. Some advocate bedrest or at least reduced activity for 12–24 h following steroid injection into a large weight-bearing joint, to improve therapeutic benefit. However, no special advice is required following aspiration alone.

Joints of patients who are anticoagulated may be aspirated. Pressure over the aspiration site is merely applied for a longer period. The procedure should be as atraumatic as possible and ideally undertaken by an experienced operator.

SPECIFIC JOINT SITES

Most joints are readily amenable to aspiration. Important exceptions are the hip, sacroiliac, spinal apophyseal and intervertebral joints, which usually require imaging control (ultrasound or fluoroscopy) and an experienced operator.

The knee

The knee is the largest synovial joint and the easiest to aspirate. Being a target joint for all major arthropathies and the commonest site for septic arthritis and pseudogout, it is by far the commonest joint to require aspiration.

A knee effusion is first evident as a loss of the medial and lateral dimples around the patella. A large effusion presents a horseshoe swelling of the suprapatellar pouch above and to either side of the patella (Fig. 16.2). Fluid may predominantly collect posteriorly as a popliteal 'cyst' but this should not be aspirated directly.

The patient should rest on a couch with their whole leg supported and relaxed. With a large, tense

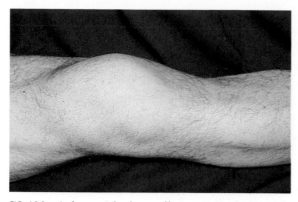

FIG 16.2 A large right knee effusion (note the smooth, horseshoe swelling above and to either side of the patella).

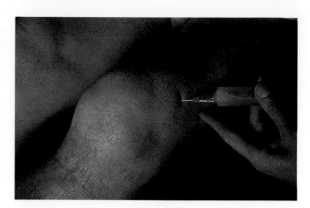

FIG 16.3 Superolateral aspiration of a large left knee effusion showing correct placement at superolateral maximum convexity of the suprapatella pouch (note the turbid SF from this patient with acute 'pseudogout').

effusion, the knee is most comfortable held in mild to moderate flexion (the 'loose-pack' position). If this is present, a soft support, such as a pillow, should be placed under the mildly flexed knee. It is important to allow the patient to relax their quadriceps to prevent the patella from being clamped down into the patellar groove. A superolateral approach is commonly used for large effusions that distend the suprapatellar pouch (Figs 16.3 and 16.4). The needle is introduced above and to the lateral side of the patella at the maximum convexity of the distended pouch, aiming downward and medially, as if to go under the posterolateral aspect of the patella. Aspiration should proceed as the needle is advanced – the distended pouch is superficial and the needle need not be introduced very far before SF is aspirated. The operator's free hand is used to tip the patella laterally and to apply pressure (Fig. 16.4), thus enlarging the target space and encouraging fluid to accumulate at the site of aspiration.

For smaller fluid collections that do not fully open up the suprapatellar reflection, a medial approach may be preferred (Fig. 16.5). The site of entry is just below the midpoint of the patella and the needle is aimed directly medially into the dimple in a line to go under the patella. Fluid is aspirated back as the needle is progressed. Synovial fluid is often found after just 1 cm of penetration and unnecessary deep introduction of the needle is thus avoided. Again, pressure is applied with the other hand to encourage fluid to the medial side (Fig. 16.5).

The wrist

Synovitis of the radiocarpal compartment results in swelling on the dorsal aspect of the wrist. The patient is positioned with the wrist and hand supported on a pillow and the wrist slightly flexed. The usual site of aspiration is the triangular space palpable between the distal radius, the scaphoid and the lunate, which is approximately in the midline just distal to the

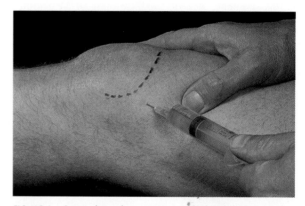

FIG 16.4 Superolateral aspiration of the left knee of a patient with rheumatoid arthritis suffering a monoarticular flare (sepsis was subsequently excluded). The patella outline is marked by the dotted line. Pressure with the operator's right hand is encouraging SF to the lateral side and facilitating the aspiration.

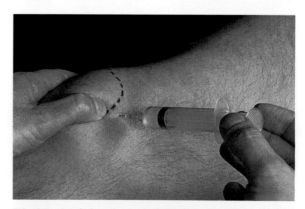

FIG 16.5 Medial aspiration of the right knee of a diabetic patient with osteoarthritis and suspected superimposed sepsis (subsequently excluded). The patellar outline is marked by the dotted line. The operator's left hand is applying pressure to encourage SF to the medial side.

radius. The needle need not be inserted very far before fluid is obtained.

The ankle

Ankle effusions present predominantly as anterior diffuse swelling, often filling the depressions in front of the malleoli. Compression with the supporting hand behind both medial and lateral malleoli presses on the posterior aspect of the capsule, encouraging SF to come forwards and increase the anterior bulge. An anterior approach is usually employed for aspiration. With the foot in moderate plantar flexion, the needle is inserted in the space between the tibia and talus, bounded medially by the tibialis anterior tendon (made prominent by asking the patient to dorsiflex the foot) and laterally by the extensor hallucis longus tendon (made prominent by asking the patient to dorsiflex and extend the big toe against resistance). The needle should be directed tangentially to the curve of the talus – a common mistake is to direct the needle too much towards the heel and thus hit the periosteum of the talus. Again, SF will often be obtained after relatively shallow penetration.

EXAMINATION AND INVESTIGATION OF SYNOVIAL FLUID

Macroscopic appearance

Normal SF contains very few cells and is clear, colourless to pale yellow, and highly viscous (Box 16.3). Only small volumes are present in a normal joint (e.g. 0–2 mL may be obtained from the largest synovial joint – the knee). In general, with increasing inflammation (Fig. 16.6), the volume increases, the total cell count rises with an increasing proportion of neutrophils (causing

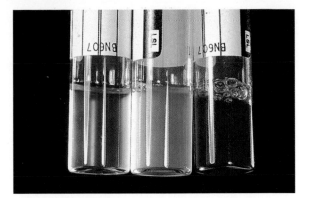

FIG 16.6　Three contrasting SF samples. The left SF is from a patient with osteoarthritis and is clear and straw coloured ('non-inflammatory'). The middle SF is from a patient with rheumatoid arthritis and is more turbid (higher cell count) and less viscous. The right SF is from a patient with acute pseudogout and shows uniform bloodstaining.

turbidity) and the viscosity reduces (principally due to protease digestion of hyaluronate). There is considerable overlap, however, between different diagnostic conditions, and the macroscopic appearance of the SF cannot be relied upon to differentiate, for example, sepsis from osteoarthritis. Frank pus or 'pyarthrosis' (due to very high neutrophil counts) always points to sepsis, but may occur with any florid synovitis (e.g. rheumatoid arthritis or acute crystal synovitis). White SF or joint 'milk' occasionally occurs in gross gout (urate crystals are white macroscopically) and rarely with cholesterol crystal deposition.

Non-uniform bloodstaining, reflecting needle trauma to synovial vessels, is common, particularly in inflammatory joint disease with friable synovial hypertrophy. Uniform bloodstaining of SF (haemarthrosis; Fig. 16.6) is most commonly seen in association with florid synovitis (e.g. pseudogout) but may also result from a bleeding diathesis or pigmented villonodular synovitis (Box 16.4). A lipid

---

BOX 16.3　SYNOVIAL FLUID APPEARANCE

- 'Non-inflammatory'
  — clear
  — straw coloured
  — high viscosity
- 'Inflammatory'
  — cloudy/turbid
  — yellow/orange
  — medium/low viscosity
  — often bloodstained
- 'Joint milk'
  — crystals (urate or cholesterol)
- 'Rice bodies'
  — small, fibrinous lumps (usually only with chronic inflammatory disease)

BOX 16.4　CAUSES OF HAEMARTHROSIS

- Trauma
- Severe inflammation, e.g.
  — infection
  — rheumatoid arthritis
  — pyrophosphate arthropathy
- Bleeding diathesis, e.g.
  — anticoagulated
  — haemophilia
  — scurvy
- Abnormal vessels, e.g.
  — haemangioma
- Pigmented villonodular synovitis (a benign synovial tumour)
- Malignant synovial/cartilage/bone tumours (rare)

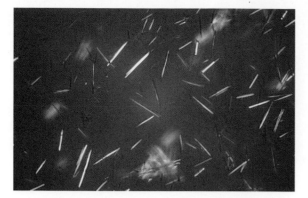

FIG 16.7 Monosodium urate crystals in SF viewed under compensated polarized light. The crystals are brightly birefringent and show a negative sign of birefringence (determined by the known optics of this particular microscope). The large size (up to 20 μm) and needle-shaped morphology are highly characteristic.

layer over bloodstained SF is pathognomonic of an intra-articular fracture.

Investigations

The two routine investigations of diagnostic importance are: (1) Gram stain and culture, and (2) polarized microscopy for crystals.

If joint infection is suspected, a sample of SF must be sent for **urgent Gram stain and culture** (Box 16.5). Placement in paired blood culture bottles, in addition to a sterile universal container, increases positive yields, especially of anaerobes. Although a positive result on Gram staining is found in over 50% of cases of adult septic arthritis (predominantly *Staph. aureus*), a negative result does not exclude sepsis. If there is a strong clinical suspicion of infection, the patient should be treated as having sepsis, with intravenous antibiotics administered pending the results of the SF, blood and other culture results.

Crystal identification is potentially problematic and is best undertaken using **compensated polarized microscopy** and **an experienced operator**. Urate (gout; Fig. 16.7) and calcium pyrophosphate (pseudogout) crystals may be seen by ordinary light microscopy but confident identification resides in their birefringence and extinction angles, in addition to their morphology. Crystal identification is best performed on fresh SF (within 2 h of collection, unrefrigerated) taken into a plain container to avoid problems of postaspiration crystallization, crystal dissolution and artefacts from tube additives. Such specialized examination is usually undertaken by the rheumatological team.

INDICATIONS AND SIDE-EFFECTS OF CONCURRENT STEROID INJECTION

The principal indication for intra-articular injection of steroid is for relief of pain and swelling from inflammatory arthritis. Steroid should not be injected if infection is suspected or the diagnosis is in doubt. Generally, injections should not be repeated more often than at 3-monthly intervals – frequent requirement often means that other treatment modalities are being underutilized. Only long-acting steroid preparations should be used. For large joints (e.g. knee, hip, ankle, glenohumeral or elbow), 40 mg of methylprednisolone or 20 mg of triamcinolone should be given; half these amounts being used for smaller joints. The patient should be warned that the joint may feel uncomfortable for 24 h and that they should avoid excessive use of the joint for that period. It may take several days before they notice any improvement in symptoms.

Potential side-effects are listed in Box 16.6. Fluorinated steroid (e.g. triamcinolone hexacetonide or triamcinolone acetonide) is particularly prone to cause permanent local skin changes and should not be used for small superficial joints. Provided appropriate sterile precautions are used, the risk of introducing sepsis is extremely small.

BOX 16.5   SYNOVIAL FLUID ANALYSIS

Microbiology
■ Urgent Gram stain
■ Culture (special media required if gonococcus, fungi or other unusual organisms suspected)
■ Ziehl–Nielson stain if TB suspected (NB: culture of synovial biopsy gives higher yield and is usually required)

Polarized light microscopy
■ Crystals

NB: SF should be sent *fresh* in *sterile plain containers*.
Inclusion of SF injected into *blood culture bottles* increases positive yield.

BOX 16.6   POTENTIAL SIDE-EFFECTS OF INTRA-ARTICULAR STEROIDS

- Flushing
  - — mainly facial
  - — self-limiting within 24–72 h
- Local skin/fat atrophy
- Local skin depigmentation
- Acute flare (predominantly with crystalline preparations due to crystal-induced synovitis)
- Infection

FURTHER READING

Dixon, A. St J. and Graber, J. 1983: *Local injection therapy in rheumatic diseases*. Basle, Switzerland: Eular.

Doherty, M., Hazleman, B., Hutton, C., Maddison, P. and Perry, D. 1992: *Rheumatology examination and injection techniques*. London: W.B. Saunders.

17

Percutaneous Needle Muscle Biopsy

INTRODUCTION

Needle quadriceps muscle biopsy is a rapid, easy technique which can be performed under local anaesthesia in an out-patient clinic, and can be subsequently repeated for follow-up purposes if necessary. This contrasts with open muscle biopsy which, although supplying large complete samples, usually requires admission to hospital, a visit to the operating theatre, and a general anaesthetic. It also results in a sizeable scar. Needle biopsy is consequently less expensive and, although offering smaller samples, can enter much deeper muscles and sample multiple sites within a muscle, which may help to reduce sample bias error. Such advantages have reduced the threshold for performing a muscle biopsy.

INDICATIONS

Patients commonly report muscle symptoms which typically include stiffness, aching, weakness and tenderness. After taking a history and completing an examination, the doctor may attribute the symptoms to a muscular disorder. However, the pathological process may not be apparent and, although serum creatine kinase estimations can be useful and electrophysiological studies helpful, these do not precisely indicate the pathological changes within the muscle (Box 17.1). Inflammatory, degenerative and inherited disorders of muscle can be identified through appropriate handling of biopsied muscle and, as a bonus, changes in blood vessels and nerves can also be assessed.

BOX 17.1   INDICATIONS FOR PERCUTANEOUS MUSCLE BIOPSY

- Muscle weakness, having excluded a neuropathic cause (possibly by neurophysiology) and myasthenia gravis
- Unexplained abnormal muscle fatigue ± muscle cramps
- Following an unexplained episode of rhabdomyolysis
- Unexplained muscle pain on exertion
- To aid the diagnosis of multisystem disease (e.g. systemic vasculitis)
- To assess effects of therapy and to exclude supervening steroid myopathy

CHOICE OF MUSCLE

Normally, the quadriceps muscle is selected. Other muscles can be biopsied by experienced operators but these should not be attempted until the operator is well versed in percutaneous needle muscle biopsy technique. Possible alternative sites are the deltoid and calf muscles; if these are used, a detailed knowledge of the relevant anatomy is required.

PROCEDURE

Before starting, one should check that:

- the patient is not on anticoagulants and does not have a bleeding tendency;

■ the patient understands the procedure and has given consent;
■ all equipment is available at hand (Box 17.2);
■ a suitably qualified assistant is available.

BOX 17.2   ITEMS REQUIRED FOR PERCUTANEOUS MUSCLE BIOPSY

■ Antiseptic skin-cleansing agent (e.g. chlorhexidine)
■ Sterile surgical gloves
■ Basic dressing pack plus additional gauze squares
■ Cotton wool balls
■ Needles
■ Steri-strips (12 × 100 mm)
■ Roll of Micropore adhesive tape (25 mm wide)
■ 4–6 in crepe bandage
■ 25 mL normal saline
■ 5 mL 2% lignocaine
■ Sterile universal container
■ 5 mL syringe
■ Scalpel blade on a small handle
■ Muscle biopsy needle (*see* Fig. 17.1)
■ Sterile towels and dressing pad

Position

The patient is made comfortable on the couch, lying supine and positioned towards the edge to allow easier access to the thigh which is to be biopsied. The vastus lateralis is commonly selected as it is easily accessible and devoid of large blood vessels and nerves. Sites of recent trauma, including injection sites and areas recently subjected to electromyography, should be avoided.

Technique

The skin entry site is selected and marked; it should be approximately the midpoint between the anterior superior iliac spine and the head of the fibula, and midway between the upper and lower surfaces of the thigh. One should be aware, at this stage, that a pressure bandage will need to be positioned around the thigh, and therefore the entry site for the biopsy on the lateral surface of the thigh should be far enough below the groin to enable the bandage to be easily wrapped around the leg. The lateral thigh approach is recommended.

The operator washes their hands and puts on surgical gloves. The thigh is cleaned with an appropriate cleansing agent, such as chlorhexidine, and the area is towelled, remembering that the superior aspect of the thigh must be covered to enable gentle

downward pressure to be applied to the thigh during the procedure without compromising sterility. Another sterile towel must be placed under the thigh.

At least 4 mL of 2% plain lignocaine is drawn up into the syringe. An orange-hubbed 25 G needle is used to infiltrate the skin and a green-hubbed 21 G needle is used to inject into the subcutaneous tissues, to and through the tensor fascia lata (i.e. to the hilt of the 21 G needle). There is no need to anaesthetize the muscle as it is remarkably pain free provided the operator is gentle.

When the area is sufficiently anaesthetized, the blade of the scalpel is inserted up to the hilt, and possibly further, depending on the degree of adipose tissue present. The blade should be maintained in a horizontal position, aiming to keep the defect in the skin as small as possible (i.e. the width of the blade and no more). The grittiness of the tensor fascia lata can often be felt as it is cut. Using the skin entry site as a pivot, the handle of the scalpel can be moved back and forth in the horizontal plane to achieve a wider incision in the fascia lata.

Using an angle of entry into the thigh similar to that used with the scalpel, the assembled biopsy needle (Fig. 17.1) is inserted into the skin incision using a gentle boring motion, passing through the subcutaneous tissues and the preformed incision in the tensor fascia lata and into the muscle. If significant resistance is felt, then there has either been failure to make a cut in the tensor fascia lata or failure to use the same tract as that created by the scalpel. Unanaesthetized muscle can be gently penetrated without discomfort to the patient. However, if muscle is stretched during the biopsy needle entry, then pain will be registered by the patient!

Once the needle is in the belly of the muscle, the introducer is removed and the trocar (cutting implement) partly withdrawn. To encourage muscle to enter the cavity of the needle, one of two techniques can be adopted:

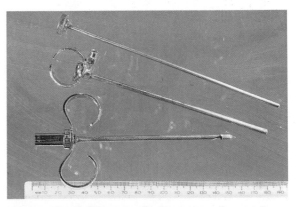

FIG 17.1   Muscle biopsy needle. From top to bottom: introducer, biopsy needle, cutting trocar.

1. With a 20 mL syringe attached to the side arm of the biopsy needle, suction can be applied; then, by closing the cutting implement, an adequate biopsy can be achieved.

2. With the needle appropriately positioned in the muscle and the aperture pointing upwards, the cutting portal is opened and the hand holding the needle is lowered towards the couch; this results (using the skin entry site as the pivot) in the cutting aperture being pressed into the overlying muscle. With one hand placed flat on the thigh, gentle downward pressure can be simultaneously applied and, if the cutting implement is then closed, a sample of muscle will be obtained.

The whole needle is withdrawn and, with the end of the scalpel, the muscle sample is removed from the needle and placed on a saline-dampened gauze swab (Fig. 17.2). Further samples can be taken as required. It is customary to take two or three biopsies, provided the procedure is well tolerated. One should remember to check the biopsy needle for any pieces of muscle that might be concealed in its nooks and crannies.

The sterile damp gauze is critical to maintenance of the muscle in a moist condition during transportation to the laboratory. The gauze swab should have been soaked in normal saline and then squeezed dry in the palm of the hand; the object is to prevent

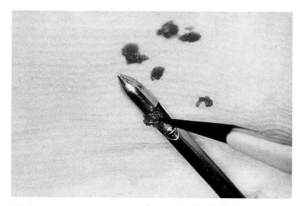

FIG 17.2   Removal of the biopsy from the port of the cutting implement.

drying but not to overhydrate and damage the muscle architecture. It is critical that the histopathologist is warned to expect the arrival of the sample and is aware of the diagnostic possibilities. The biopsy and gauze are sent to the laboratory in a sealed universal container.

The wound is then cleaned and dried. Steri-strips are applied to the small skin defect and a pad is applied and fixed with strips of Micropore tape. Finally, a 4–6 in crepe bandage is applied to the thigh.

Laboratory handling

Muscle biopsies need to be received in the laboratory within 2 h of the biopsy being taken. Not all histopathology laboratories will have the expertise to handle muscle that has been appropriately and adeptly obtained. Therefore, as pointed out earlier, previous liaison with the laboratory is essential and immediate transportation is mandatory. It takes at least 1 h, after arrival of the sample in the Histopathology Department, for processing to occur, and samples cannot adequately be stored overnight. Samples must not be placed in formalin as this causes both shrinkage artefacts and, more importantly, inactivation of the enzymes vital to histochemistry.

It must be remembered that the histology of calf muscles is different from that of the quadriceps in that type 1 fibres predominate. Unless one has clearly indicated the site of the biopsy, the histopathologist may report type 2 atrophy – which is the normal finding in calf muscle!

AFTERCARE

Biopsy sites usually heal rapidly without complications; the bandage can be removed at the end of the day of the procedure, the pad on the following evening and the Steri-strips on the third postoperative day. There is no need for the patient to rest on the day of the biopsy but vigorous activity, such as sport, is probably best avoided.

18

Fine-Needle Aspiration for Cytology

INTRODUCTION

The use of fine-needle aspiration to obtain a diagnostic, cytological specimen was first advocated in the UK and the USA in the late 1920s and early 1930s. However, the technique, though simple to perform, did not flourish until the 1950s and 1960s when it began to be practised successfully in Europe, particularly in Sweden and Holland. Since then, it has gradually been taken up elsewhere and now forms part of the diagnostic service of most hospitals.

The technique is applicable to almost any palpable mass and, with the aid of various radiological imaging procedures, is now being used successfully to obtain cytological samples from deep-seated lesions, for example lung masses and impalpable lesions such as those detected mammographically in Breast Screening Programmes. Its main advantages are high patient acceptability, low cost, reliability, rapidity, high diagnostic yield and low risk of serious complications. Thus, it is being used with increasing frequency, not only for hospital in-patients, but also, importantly, in out-patient clinics and GP surgeries. Its use has largely replaced frozen section in the diagnosis of tumours, thereby allowing a preoperative diagnosis and reducing time spent under general anaesthetic. The main disadvantage of fine-needle aspiration cytology (FNAC) is that its success is directly related to the skill and experience of the personnel involved in taking the specimen and interpreting the smears.

There is continuing debate about who should perform the aspiration, with a large body of opinion advocating that this, together with the preparation of smears and cytological interpretation, should all be performed by the same person, namely the cytopathologist, who thereby rapidly gains and maintains a high level of expertise. However, as this is not routine practice in many centres, where the aspirator is usually a clinician, it is essential that there is regular contact between clinicians and cytopathologists to ensure that the inadequacy rate is kept to a minimum and reasons for inadequate smears are identified and eliminated.

INDICATIONS

As mentioned above, almost any easily palpable lesion can be aspirated. Thus, this technique is used commonly in the investigation of skin and subcutaneous masses, palpable breast lumps, thyroid nodules and lymphadenopathy. The technique described below for superficial, palpable lesions can also be modified for impalpable and deep-seated lesions, such as lung and hepatic masses, using various imaging techniques. In all cases, aspiration is directed at a target lesion and therefore is not suitable as a screening test for possible malignancy unless such a lesion has been identified.

PRELIMINARY CONSIDERATIONS AND PATIENT PREPARATION

As with any practical procedure, some apprehension on the part of the patient is to be expected and may be alleviated to some extent by taking time to explain the nature and purpose of the investigation. Usually, neither prebiopsy sedation nor local anaesthesia are required. Indeed, the injection of local anaesthetic is often as painful as the procedure itself, whose main discomfort occurs during the initial skin puncture, the deeper tissues being less sensitive in the vast majority of cases. Furthermore, the injection of local anaesthetic may make the lesion difficult to feel. If local anaesthetic is considered desirable, for example when performing FNAC on a child, then a topical application to produce surface anaesthesia is the method of choice. If this is not available, then local anaesthetic should be injected into the skin and immediate subcutaneous tissue only. In certain situations, particularly if performing FNAC on a child, then local anaesthesia, sedation or even general anaesthesia may be considered.

The procedure is ideally performed with the patient lying supine on an examination couch, although this may not always be possible, as with a patient having severe orthopnoea, in which case a semi-prone position may have to be adopted. Slight modifications may be made, depending on the site of the target lesion. For example, thyroid lesions are often more easily palpated if the cervical spine is slightly extended by placing a pillow beneath the patient's shoulders.

TECHNIQUE

BOX 18.1   STEP-BY-STEP GUIDE TO FNAC

- Explain the procedure to the patient
- Ensure necessary equipment is to hand and label slides
- Position the patient (preferably supine) and relocate target lesion
- Clean skin with disinfectant wipe
- Immobilize lesion with non-dominant hand
- Insert needle through the skin, ensuring it is in the lesion
- Apply negative pressure
- Make multiple passes through the lesion without withdrawing the needle through the skin and while maintaining negative pressure
- Release negative pressure
- Withdraw needle and instruct patient or assistant to apply pressure to the puncture site
- Remove needle from syringe and draw air into syringe
- Reconnect needle and gently express specimen onto labelled glass slide
- Prepare smears and air dry or wet fix as necessary

Equipment

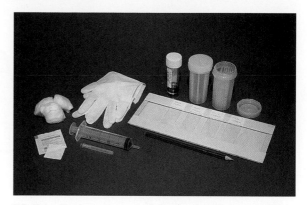

FIG 18.1   Equipment required for fine-needle aspiration.

Needles

Standard disposable 21–25 G needles are generally suitable, with the finest (25 G) being recommended for children and for the aspiration of particularly sensitive areas such as the eyelids. It should be stressed that thicker needles offer no advantage in obtaining a better yield and may, in fact, be disadvantageous as they are more likely to cause bleeding and thereby produce an inadequate sample. Needle length is obviously an important consideration and should be borne in mind, particularly when aspirating breast lesions which are often deeper than indicated by palpation. Most disposable needles have a translucent plastic hub which allows the recovery of tissue, blood or other fluid to be checked.

Syringes

Disposable plastic syringes (10 or 20 mL) are ideal, the choice being one of personal preference and related to convenience, comfort and ease of manipulation rather than the minimal differences in negative pressure achievable.

Syringe holder

Unless performing aspiration without suction the Zajdela technique, (see section below), the use of a syringe holder, although a matter of personal preference, is recommended as it leaves one hand completely free to locate and stabilize the target lesion.

Slides

Glass slides with frosted ends are recommended as these may be readily labelled in pencil immediately before the procedure. At least two are required, although as many smears should be made as possible.

Fixatives

Both air-dried and wet-fixed smears may be prepared. The latter may be placed in a Coplin jar containing 70–90% alcohol or other fixative, or may be spray fixed, although spray fixation has the disadvantage of tending to push the cells to the edge of the slide unless applied with caution.

Other

Sterile containers containing special culture or transport media should be available for washing out the needle and syringe if a cell suspension is to be prepared. Empty sterile containers should also be on hand to allow submission of material for microbiological examination if infection is suspected clinically or if purulent material is unexpectedly obtained at aspiration. Alcohol-based skin disinfectant swabs are all that is required for skin disinfection in most cases, although more elaborate means may be preferred in immunosuppressed patients. Cotton wool or gauze swabs are required for applying pressure to the puncture site after the procedure, and plasters should be available. Local anaesthetic should not be required but, again, should be available. Gloves are probably not necessary but most operators would prefer to wear them.

Finally, although the procedure can be performed by one person, it is an advantage to have an assistant to reassure the patient, apply pressure to the puncture site after the aspiration and help make the smears and dry the slides (see below).

Examining the patient

Before attempting an aspiration, the target lesion should be repalpated and any changes since previous examinations noted. The lesion may be more difficult to locate when the patient is supine; this is particularly so for cervical and supraclavicular lesions, and minor adjustments of the neck should be made until the aspirator is confident that the lesion has been located and can be held immobile for the procedure. It is most important that the patient should be in a comfortable position during the procedure and one which allows the operator unhindered access.

Performing the aspiration

First, the skin is cleaned with a disinfectant wipe and the mass relocated and stabilized with the index finger and thumb of the non-dominant hand. The syringe holder with attached needle and syringe is then taken up and the needle advanced through the skin and into the lesion. Usually, the needle is introduced in such a direction that the shortest route is

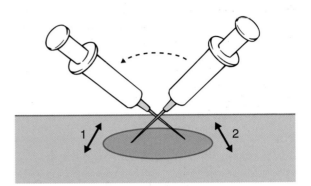

FIG 18.2 Performing the aspiration. Once the needle tip has entered the lesion, suction is applied and the needle is moved backwards and forward within the lesion (1), rotating the needle to cut with the bevel. The needle is then withdrawn from the lesion and reinserted at a different angle (2) to obtain further biopsies from different sites.

taken between the skin surface and the lesion. However, there are certain exceptions. For example, if the lesion is a small, superficial one, then the needle may be bent to a 45° angle instead and the lesion approached from the side and aspirated from its deep surface. Similarly, if the skin overlying the lesion is particularly sensitive, for example periareolar skin, then the lesion may be pushed to one side if possible and, again, the aspiration performed via adjacent, less sensitive skin. It is important that the aspirator is confident that the lesion has been entered; aspiration of adjacent, particularly superficial tissue is an important cause of false negative reports.

Once the needle tip has entered the lesion, suction is applied and the needle is moved backwards and forwards within the lesion, rotating the needle to cut with the bevel. Maintaining negative pressure, the needle is then withdrawn just out of the lesion but remains beneath the skin surface and is reinserted at a slightly different angle. In this way, multiple passes can be made through the lesion using one skin puncture.

While performing these actions, the aspirator's attention should be divided between the patient's face for signs of distress and monitoring the needle hub for aspirated material. No material will usually enter the syringe itself, except in the case of cyst fluids, very bloody aspirations or high-volume specimens such as abscesses or necrotic areas.

Blood impairs the cytological detail of subsequent films and the degree of trauma/bloody taps is proportional to the time taken over the procedure. The aim is to become sufficiently adept so that FNA is performed rapidly. If blood is seen in the hub of the needle, the aspiration should be discontinued. Further passes may need to be made in adjacent, non-traumatized areas. Even after an adequate FNA, no material will be seen in the needle hub or syringe as it is contained within the metal cylinder of the needle. It is only when material is expressed onto the slides that adequacy of the technique can be assessed. If the material appears inadequate and the patient has tolerated the procedure, then FNA may be repeated.

The aspiration is completed by first releasing the negative pressure, then withdrawing the needle from the skin. The patient or an assistant is then asked to apply pressure to the puncture site using a piece of cotton wool or gauze while the aspirator prepares the smears (*see* section below). The whole procedure should only take a few seconds.

The Zajdela technique

Negative pressure plays only a minor role in obtaining a sample compared with the cutting effect of the advancing, sharp needle tip. An alternative technique is to dispense with the syringe and hold the needle directly with the fingertips, moving it backwards and forwards within the lesion as before. The advantage of this technique is that the lesion can be felt with more precision, making it especially effective for aspirating tiny lesions. Another important advantage is that the sample obtained is less bloody, making it particularly suited for sampling lesions where this is often a problem, for example in the thyroid. Its main disadvantage is that the cell yield is less than with aspiration although adequate yields should be obtained with experience, and in some centres it is the method of choice for most lesions.

PREPARING THE SMEARS

Preparing good smears is an important part of the technique and failure to do so is a common reason for inadequate reports. The type of smears (i.e. air dried or wet fixed) is dictated partly by the lesion

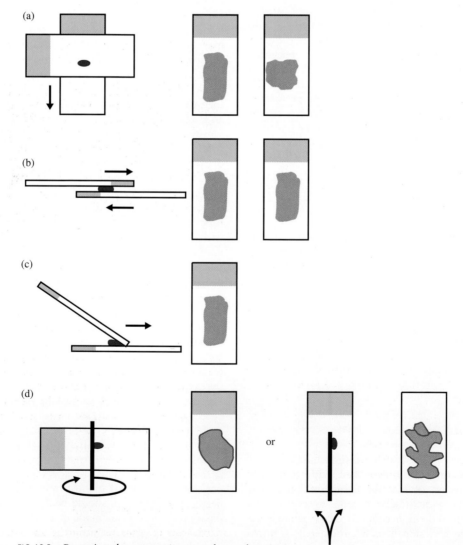

FIG 18.3   Preparing the smears (see text for explanation).

itself and partly by local laboratory preferences; if in any doubt, the laboratory should first be contacted. Additionally, in some units, after preparing the smears, the needle may be washed in special transport medium and the sample examined after cytocentrifugation. Indeed, in some units, particularly where the aspirators are not used to making cytological smears and do not follow proper fixation methods, the entire aspirate is placed in such media. However, these cytocentrifuge preparations may produce artefacts and are generally inferior to good smears prepared at the time of aspiration.

Spreading the smears

The material is expressed from the needle by first removing the syringe, drawing some air into it, replacing the needle, then gently expressing one drop onto a slide. If a large sample has been obtained, then further drops may be divided between several slides. Some aspirators may prefer to perform the whole procedure with a few millilitres of air in the syringe to avoid having to remove and replace the needle at this point. If the Zajdela method has been used, a syringe is now attached to the needle to express its contents. It is important to express the contents gently with the needle tip touching the surface of the slide, and not to spray the specimen onto the surface from above as this will give an unsatisfactory preparation.

A number of methods are available to spread the droplet so obtained. All address the problem of obtaining a thin layer of material on the slide to allow for rapid drying for air-dried preparations without causing artefacts due to excess pressure (Fig. 18.3).

(a) With the droplet towards the labelled end of the lower slide, a second slide is gently lowered onto it. This slide is orientated with its long axis perpendicular to the first but with the two flat surfaces parallel. The droplet is spread by moving the upper slide along the long axis of the lower, towards its unlabelled end. Thus, two smeared slides are produced.

(b) Again, the droplet is placed towards the labelled end of the lower slide and the second slide is gently lowered onto it, this time with their long axes parallel and such that the droplet touches the upper slide close to its labelled end. The smears are made by drawing the two labelled ends away from each other such that the smear spreads along the long axes of both slides.

(c) The droplet is placed towards the labelled end of a slide. The second slide is lowered onto the first at a 45° angle and moved 'backwards' (i.e. away from the subsequent direction it will take to make the smear) to touch the drop which spreads out along the line of contact of the two slides. The smear is made by moving the upper slide away

from the label, maintaining the 45° angle. Thus, one smear is produced per droplet.

(d) In this method, the smear is produced by placing the droplet in the centre of a slide and spreading it out using a pipette or needle. Again, this method produces one smear per droplet.

Whichever method is used, it is essential that no excess downward pressure is applied, nor that surface tension is allowed to squash or distort the cells making the slides uninterpretable.

Fixation

If air-dried smears are required, then, immediately after spreading, the slides should be waved in air or in front of a fan to allow rapid drying. If a hair-drier is used, it should only be used on a cold setting as hot air will produce artefacts.

For wet fixation, the smears should be placed in fixative, or have this applied, immediately after spreading to prevent air-drying artefacts.

COMPLICATIONS

BOX 18.2   COMPLICATIONS OF FINE-NEEDLE ASPIRATION

- Pain
- Haemorrhage/haematoma
- Vasovagal attacks
- Tracheal puncture (with thyroid nodules)
- Pneumothorax (with chest lesions)
- Infection

Pain

When performed competently and efficiently, the procedure should not be unduly painful and should be only marginally or no more painful than venepuncture. However, the skin may be particularly sensitive in some areas and the technique may need to be modified as mentioned previously. Another example in which the procedure may be more painful is if the needle encounters periosteum, as may happen during aspiration of breast masses. Appreciation of the local anatomy and entering the mass at a slight angle may help. Similarly, as aspiration through skeletal muscle is painful, thyroid nodules are best aspirated with the neck slightly extended, the sternocleidomastoid muscle pushed laterally and the needle angled toward the midline.

Haemorrhage/haematoma

Occasionally, especially during aspiration of breast masses, a superficial vein may be punctured. This not only results in an inadequate, bloodstained sample, but also in a haematoma, the extent of which is minimized by applying pressure to the area after the needle is removed.

Vasovagal attack

As with many practical procedures, patients may faint. The problem is minimized if the patient is supine during the procedure but if this is not possible, for other reasons, it is probably advisable to have an assistant on hand.

Tracheal puncture

The trachea may be entered during thyroid aspiration and is recognized at the time by air entering the syringe, and on the smears by the presence of respiratory epithelial cells or, occasionally, haematopoietic cells if ossified cartilage is aspirated. There are no adverse clinical consequences.

Rare complications

Pneumothorax has rarely been described during aspiration of breast masses and is recognized by sudden thoracic pain without dyspnoea. It is unlikely to be severe and may be avoided by entering the lesion with the needle tangential rather than perpendicular to the skin surface. Infections are extremely rare, even following transrectal aspiration of the prostate. Likewise, implantation of malignant cells in the needle tract, often cited as an objection to FNA, has been found to be extremely rare in follow-up studies.

PROBLEMS WITH SMEARS

Inadequate smears

This is the most common problem encountered, particularly with inexperienced aspirators. There are several reasons, as outlined below:

- *Insufficient material.* The likelihood of this being so is minimized by performing multiple aspirates, and ensuring that the needle is actually within the lesion. Occasionally, only necrotic material is obtained. Again, this should not be a problem if multiple areas are sampled.
- *Heavily bloodstained smears.* These are often impossible to interpret. They are a particular

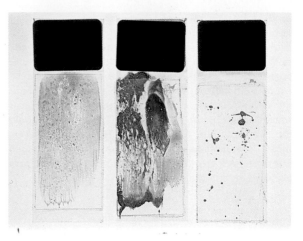

FIG 18.4 Examples of smears: left, an adequate smear; centre, too thick; right, specimen sprayed onto the slide.

problem with thyroid aspirates and prevention requires a more gentle approach to the procedure, or even adoption of the Zajdela technique.
- *Smearing and fixation artefacts.* These are a common problem, directly related to the experience of the operator, and can only be prevented by frequent practice and feedback from microscopic examination. An example of a well-spread smear is given in Fig. 18.4. Two inadequate smears are shown for comparison. The central smear is far too thick, whereas that on the right is the result of the sample being sprayed onto the glass from above. In neither case was the cytological detail sufficient for assessment.

Interpretation of results

Occasionally, unexpected results may be obtained and although the technique has a high sensitivity and specificity, false positive and negative results do occur. For this reason, it is essential that the person reporting the smear is provided with as much clinical information as possible in order for it to be interpreted in the correct clinical context. For this reason, regular interdisciplinary meetings between clinicians and cytopathologists are recommended.

FURTHER READING

Stanley, M.W. and Lowhagen, T. 1993: *Fine needle aspiration of palpable masses.* Boston, MA: Butterworth-Heinemann.

19

Cardiopulmonary Resuscitation

INTRODUCTION

The aims of cardiopulmonary resuscitation (CPR) are to maintain, and ultimately restore, the breathing and circulation in a patient in whom either, or both, have suddenly ceased. Cardiopulmonary resuscitation is frequently divided into 'basic' and 'advanced' life support. Basic life support aims to maintain the patient's ventilation and circulation until the necessary drugs and equipment (and the skills to use them) can be made available for advanced life support to begin.

It is generally agreed that there should be a uniform approach to the teaching and implementation of basic and advanced life support. With this objective in mind, the European Resuscitation Council was established in 1990 and the basic and advanced life support guidelines presented in this chapter are based upon the recommendations of the Basic Life Support Working Party/Group of the European Resuscitation Council (1992, 1993) and the Advanced Life Support Working Party of the European Resuscitation Council (1992).

BASIC LIFE SUPPORT

Time is of the essence in performing effective cardiopulmonary resuscitation – any delay in the commencement of CPR reduces the likelihood of a successful outcome (Box 19.1). It is therefore imperative that immediate aid is given by anyone who witnesses a patient's collapse. A flow chart summarizing basic life support is shown in Fig. 19.1.

BOX 19.1   FACTORS ASSOCIATED WITH IMPROVED SURVIVAL FROM CPR

- Witnessed cardiac arrest
- CPR commenced by a bystander
- Arrhythmia is ventricular fibrillation
- Defibrillation is performed early in arrest

The patient's unresponsiveness is confirmed by gently shaking him/her and asking loudly, 'Are you alright?' If there is no response, immediately shout for help or send a bystander to call for assistance. The patient must not be left alone.

The patient's airway is opened by loosening any clothing around the neck, opening the mouth and removing any obstructions such as food or loose dentures. Well-fitting dentures may help to seal the mouth during ventilation and should be left in place. With one hand on the forehead, tilt the head backwards and, using two fingers of the other hand, lift the chin (Fig. 19.2). These actions will lift the tongue from the back of the throat.

Once the airway is clear, lean forwards to listen at the patient's mouth for breath sounds and feel for exhaled air on one's cheek while carefully observing the patient's chest for any movement. At the same time, assess the patient's circulation by palpating the carotid pulse. Observation is continued for 5 s before proceeding.

If the patient is breathing, he/she is rolled into the recovery position (Fig. 19.3) unless this may lead to further injury. The aim of the recovery position is to prevent obstruction of the airway by the tongue and

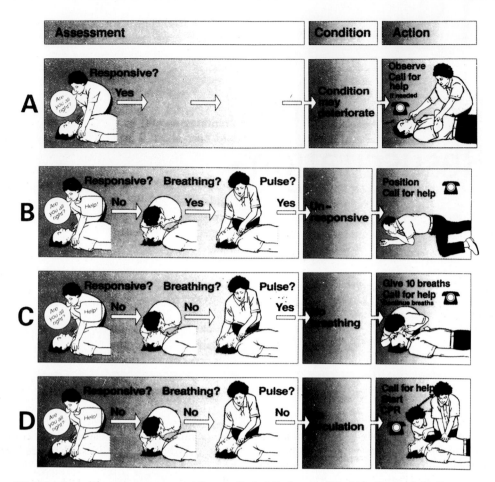

FIG 19.1 Basic life support summary. Source: Basic Life Support Working Party of the European Resuscitation Council. 1992: Guidelines for basic life support. *Resuscitation* 24, p. 110.

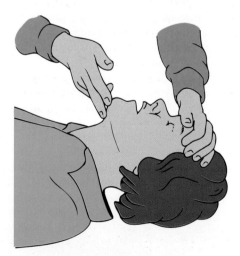

FIG 19.2 Head tilt and chin lift.

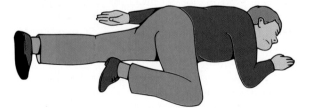

FIG 19.3 Recovery position.

reduce the chance that the patient will aspirate gastric contents. Once in a stable position, observe the patient continuously until help arrives.

If no spontaneous breathing is observed but a carotid pulse is felt, expired air respiration is commenced. With the patient lying supine, pinch the nose and while still tilting the head, lift the chin so that the mouth opens slightly. The resuscitator seals their lips around the patient's mouth and exhales for about 2 s, watching the chest to see that it rises. Then, the resuscitator moves their mouth away and watches for the patient's chest to fall while taking another breath in.

The process is repeated a total of 10 times. At this stage, one may stop briefly to obtain assistance or telephone for help if no-one else has been available to do so. Return to the patient as soon as possible to reassess them and, if necessary, continue expired air

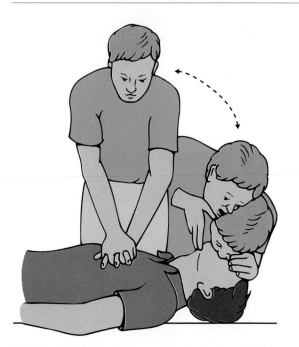

FIG 19.4   Chest compression and expired air respiration.

The mechanism by which chest compression maintains blood flow remains uncertain. The heart may be directly compressed between the sternum and vertebrae while changes in intrathoracic pressure transmitted to extrathoracic arteries may provide a vascular gradient which drives the circulation.

To achieve full neurological recovery, CPR must maintain a cerebral blood flow of at least 20% of normal. However, the ability of chest compression to provide adequate cerebral perfusion appears to decline rapidly with any delay between the onset of the arrest and the commencement of CPR (Safar, 1984). This emphasizes the need for prompt action during a cardiac arrest.

Initiation of CPR can lead to a spontaneous recovery of the patient's breathing or circulation. If not, chest compression and ventilation should be continued. Once breathing and circulation are being maintained artificially, it is important to make the personnel and facilities for delivering advanced life support available rapidly in order to attempt to restore the patient's own breathing and circulation

respiration. Check the patient's pulse and repeat this check after every 10 breaths.

If one cannot detect spontaneous breathing and a carotid pulse during the initial assessment of the patient, commence full basic life support. With the patient lying supine on a firm surface, the patient's airway is opened, two expired air ventilations are given and chest compression is started (Fig. 19.4).

Place the heel of one hand in the middle of the lower half of the patient's sternum – this should be two finger-breadths above the xiphisternum. Then place the heel of the other hand over the first, interlocking the fingers. Lean directly over the patient so that the arms are straight and press directly downwards, depressing the sternum by 4–5 cm. Keeping the hands in position, release the pressure and repeat the chest compression at a rate of 80 compressions/min. The time taken for each chest compression should equal the time taken to release the pressure. Every 15 chest compressions are followed by two ventilations.

Until quite recently it was advised that, if two rescuers are present, one rescuer should perform chest compression while the other performs expired air expiration at a ratio of 5:1. It is now recommended that one rescuer alternately performs both chest compression and expired air respiration (at a ratio of 15:2), leaving the second rescuer free to obtain help. When the first rescuer becomes tired, the second rescuer should take over. In the hospital setting, if a full cardiac arrest team is present, there is, of course, no need for just one person to perform both chest compression and expired air respiration.

ADVANCED LIFE SUPPORT

The most important aim of advanced life support is the identification, and subsequent correction, of cardiac rhythm abnormalities. There are four arrhythmias that occur in cardiac arrest: ventricular fibrillation, pulseless ventricular tachycardia, asystole and electromechanical dissociation. The ECG appearance of each arrhythmia is illustrated in Fig. 19.5.

One should be familiar with the types of cardiac defibrillator that one is likely to encounter in the working environment (Box 19.2). Within hospitals, manual defibrillators are the most commonly used. Manual defibrillators require the operator to diagnose the cardiac rhythm (displayed on an oscilloscope screen either via electrodes or via the defibrillator paddles when placed on the chest), to select the appropriate energy level for the DC shock and to choose when to deliver it.

In the community, ambulance crews and GPs more commonly use automatic and semi-automatic ('advisory') defibrillators. With both types of device, adhesive pads are positioned on the patient's chest

BOX 19.2   TYPES OF DEFIBRILLATOR

▪ Manual: operator must diagnose arrhythmia and decide when DC shock is appropriate
▪ Semi-automatic ('advisory'): defibrillator diagnoses arrhythmia but operator must authorize defibrillation
▪ Automatic: defibrillator diagnoses arrhythmia and delivers DC shock if appropriate

Ventricular fibrillation

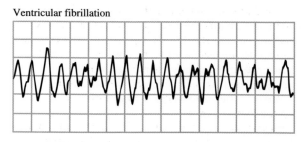

Ventricular tachycardia

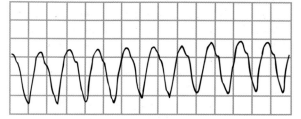

Asystole

Electromechanical dissociation

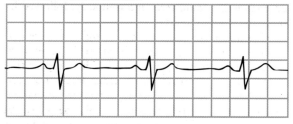

FIG 19.5   The ECG appearances of various arrhythmias.

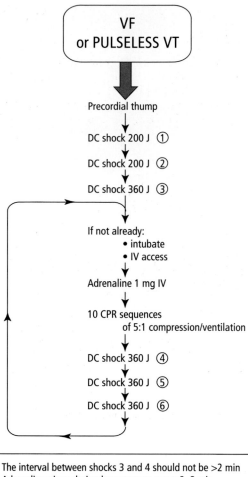

FIG 19.6   Management algorithm for ventricular fibrillation (VF) or pulseless ventricular tachycardia (VT). Source: Advanced Life Support Working Party of the European Resuscitation Council. 1992: Guidelines for advanced life support. *Resuscitation* 24, p. 115.

which allow the defibrillator both to analyse the cardiac rhythm and to deliver DC shocks as appropriate. Once an automatic defibrillator determines that a DC shock is appropriate, it will deliver it after displaying a warning to stand clear. Semi-automatic defibrillators will advise if a DC shock is required but the operator must authorize defibrillation by pressing a button.

Ventricular fibrillation/pulseless ventricular tachycardia

Ventricular fibrillation (VF) is the most frequent initial arrhythmia causing cardiac arrest. Pulseless ventricular tachycardia (VT), which may precede VF, is encountered far less commonly in its own right. The management of both arrhythmias, shown as an algorithm in Fig. 19.6, is identical. In treating these

conditions, time is of the essence. For this reason, a precordial thump should be given immediately – to do so may restore an effective rhythm in 2% of cases of VF, and up to 40% of VT cases if given within 30 s.

If a precordial thump does not restore an effective rhythm, electrical defibrillation must be performed (Box 19.3). Before any attempts at defibrillation are made, any glyceryl trinitrate (GTN) patch that may be on the patient must be removed to prevent burns. Permanent pacemakers are not a contraindication to defibrillation, but care should be taken to try to place the paddles at least 15 cm from the generator box.

The standard paddle positions are shown in Fig. 19.7. To improve electrical conduction, electrode jelly

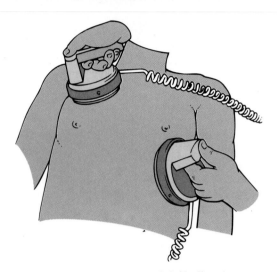

FIG 19.7 Paddle positions (manual defibrillator).

or gel pads must be placed on the skin under the paddles and pressure applied. Care must be taken to avoid spreading electrode jelly over the skin between the two paddles as this can conduct current and lead to a 'short circuit'. Some gel pads can withstand multiple DC shocks while others must be replaced after a single shock. It is essential to know what is available at one's workplace hospital.

It is the responsibility of the person operating the defibrillator to ensure that nobody is in contact with the patient or the bed so, before delivering a DC shock, everyone must be warned to stand clear. Deliver three DC shocks in rapid succession, at energies of 200 J, 200 J and then 360 J. There should be only a brief pause between each shock to recharge the defibrillator and assess the patient's rhythm and/or pulse. If all three shocks can be delivered rapidly (i.e. in less than 45 s), it is not necessary to resume basic life support between each one.

If, despite three shocks, the patient remains in VF/pulseless VT, establish intravenous access. The external jugular vein is often easily visible but a large antecubital vein is acceptable. Although the central route allows drugs to reach the central circulation more rapidly, gaining central venous access is more hazardous, especially following thrombolysis. When drugs are given peripherally, they should be flushed with 20 mL of isotonic saline.

Intubate the patient if this has not already been done. An alternative route of drug administration is via the endotracheal tube, but this is not ideal and should be avoided whenever possible. If the endotracheal route is used, drugs are given at two to three times their intravenous doses, diluted to 10 mL in isotonic saline, and drug administration is followed by five ventilations.

Attempts at endotracheal intubation and intravenous access should not delay basic life support for more than 15 s. If the attempts are unsuccessful, they should be deferred until after the next set of DC shocks. Whether the attempts succeed or not, chest compression and ventilation are recommenced at a ratio of 5:1 for a total of 10 sequences.

If possible, administer 1 mg of adrenaline intravenously, and followed with a further three DC shocks, each at an energy of 360 J. It is a common misconception that adrenaline should be given time to circulate before the shocks are given. As the effects of the adrenaline are chiefly to improve cerebral and myocardial blood flow, rather than to aid defibrillation, there is nothing to gain (and potentially much to lose) by delaying further shocks.

If a satisfactory rhythm has still not been restored and intubation or intravenous access has not been achieved, these procedures should be reattempted. Again, no more than 15 s should elapse before basic life support recommences and a further 1 mg of adrenaline is administered intravenously, followed by three more DC shocks.

No longer than 2 or 3 min should be taken to complete each 'loop', and adrenaline is given each time. The loop is repeated until either a perfusing rhythm has been obtained or it is decided that continued CPR would be inappropriate. If the patient remains in VF, consideration should be given to changing the paddle positions to anteroposterior or to changing the defibrillator itself.

After every third loop, antiarrhythmic agents such as lignocaine, bretylium or amiodarone, or potassium, calcium or magnesium salts may be administered, although evidence of benefit is questionable.

Adequate ventilation should avoid respiratory acidosis, but a marked metabolic acidosis can occur during a prolonged (more than 20 min) cardiac arrest. The routine use of an alkalizing agent, such as sodium bicarbonate, cannot be recommended because intracellular acidosis can paradoxically worsen. Sodium bicarbonate has not been shown to improve outcome.

Asystole

The management algorithm for asystole is shown in Fig. 19.8. Following a precordial thump, it is important positively to identify the rhythm as asystole. Sometimes VF is misdiagnosed as asystole, perhaps because of misinterpretation of the ECG, faulty

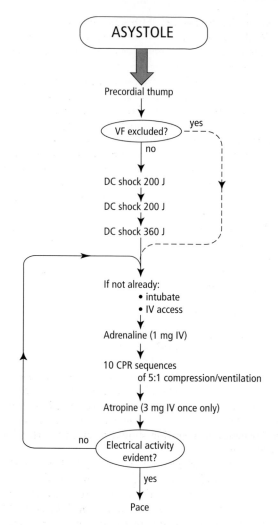

FIG 19.8 Management algorithm for asystole. Source: Advanced Life Support Working Party of the European Resuscitation Council. 1992: Guidelines for advanced life support. *Resuscitation* 24, p. 118.

equipment or an inappropriately low-gain setting on the monitor. *If there is the slightest doubt* about whether the rhythm is asystole or VF, three DC shocks at energies of 200 J, 200 J and 360 J are administered to avoid missing a potentially reversible arrhythmia. After the shocks, or if asystole can confidently be diagnosed at the outset, intubate the patient and obtain intravenous access as described earlier.

Adrenaline (1 mg) is given intravenously, followed by 10 cycles of chest compression and ventilation at a ratio of 5:1. Following this, an intravenous dose of atropine (3 mg), given once, will block vagal tone.

The loop is repeated and basic life support continued, giving repeated doses of adrenaline. If the patient remains asystolic after three cycles, high-dose adrenaline (5 mg intravenously) may be given. If electrical activity (as evidenced by P waves or occasional QRS complexes) is apparent, pacing should be considered. Either a transvenous pacing wire or transthoracic pacing can be used. Transvenous pacing is more effective but requires the appropriate skills to perform. If the patient is being paced transthoracically, ensure that this is providing an effective circulation by monitoring the pulse and blood pressure.

Electromechanical dissociation

Electromechanical dissociation (EMD) is the failure of the heart to circulate blood effectively, despite showing evidence of electrical activity (QRS complexes on the ECG). A number of potentially reversible causes are recognized and it is important to attempt to identify an underlying cause and treat it where possible (Box 19.4).

If a specific cause cannot be found, then the EMD should be treated according to the management algorithm in Fig. 19.9. Intubate the patient and establish intravenous access if not done already and administer adrenaline (1 mg) intravenously. Ten cycles of chest compression and ventilation are

---

BOX 19.4   CAUSES OF ELECTROMECHANICAL DISSOCIATION AND THEIR MANAGEMENT

Cause	*Management*
■ Cardiac tamponade	■ Pericardiocentesis
■ Drug overdose	■ Depends upon drug(s) taken ■ Discuss with nearest poisons unit
■ Electrolyte disturbance	■ Correction of electrolyte abnormalities
■ Hypothermia	■ Rewarming
■ Hypovolaemia	■ Replacement of fluid losses as appropriate (e.g. colloid infusion or blood transfusion)
■ Pulmonary embolism	■ Anticoagulation ■ Consider thrombolysis or pulmonary embolectomy
■ Tension pneumothorax	■ Chest drain

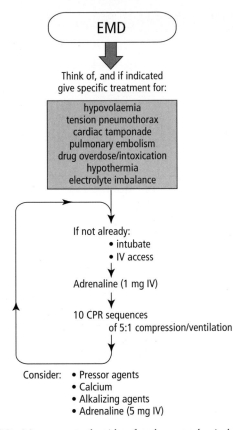

FIG 19.9 Management algorithm for electromechanical dissociation (EMD). Source: Advanced Life Support Working Party of the European Resuscitation Council. 1992: Guidelines for advanced life support. *Resuscitation* **24**, p. 120.

performed (at a ratio of 5:1), and the loop is repeated as shown in Fig. 19.9, while always looking specifically for a treatable cause.

High-dose adrenaline (5 mg intravenously), alkalizing agents, calcium and pressor agents can be given but there is no firm evidence for recommending their routine use.

CONDUCTING THE ARREST

Disorganization is commonly encountered during a cardiac arrest, especially with a poorly trained and inexperienced arrest team. During a medical emergency, rational decision making and prompt action are essential.

One person, usually the most experienced present, must take overall control of the situation from the outset. The team leader must be capable of diagnosing arrhythmias swiftly and, like all members of the arrest team, must be familiar with the basic and advanced life support guidelines, although this is often not the case: in one study, 29 out of the 30 doctors examined were found to lack basic knowl-

edge and skills (David and Prior-Willeard, 1993).

While diagnosing the arrhythmias and taking decisions accordingly, the team leader must direct the other team members by giving clear instructions to specified individuals. Ideally, one member of the team should perform chest compression (swapping with others when tired), one should be responsible for defibrillation, one should maintain oxygenation by ventilating and/or intubating the patient, one should obtain intravenous access and one should be responsible for drawing up the necessary drugs. Another team member should keep a record of the events, and count the seconds (audibly) whenever CPR is interrupted for intubation or defibrillation.

The team leader should also decide when further resuscitation appears futile and, with the rest of the team's agreement, when to terminate resuscitation efforts. Some guidance on when it is appropriate to stop CPR is given later in the chapter.

POSTARREST CARE

If resuscitation is successful, the patient is transferred to an intensive care or coronary care unit. Continued care of the patient's airway and breathing is important. In particular, if a patient's conscious level is diminished, consideration should be given to artificial ventilation.

Blood urea and electrolytes are checked, and a 12-lead ECG and chest X-ray are performed. The patient's vital signs and urine output should be frequently checked and charted. Continuous ECG monitoring is mandatory so that any further arrhythmias can be treated appropriately. Pulse oximetry may be helpful but provides no information about CO_2 concentration or acid–base balance, so one should ensure that arterial blood gas analysis is performed at regular intervals (Box 19.5).

DO NOT FORGET THE PATIENT'S RELATIVES FOLLOWING A CARDIAC ARREST. ARRANGEMENTS MUST BE MADE TO SPEAK TO THEM AS SOON AS POSSIBLE AFTER THE ARREST.

BOX 19.5 POSTRESUSCITATION CARE

Check
■ Urea and electrolytes
■ 12-lead ECG
■ Chest X-ray
■ Arterial blood gases

Monitor
■ Vital signs
■ Urine output
■ ECG
■ Arterial blood gases/pulse oximetry

TRAUMA DURING CPR

Although it can be life saving, CPR also has the potential to cause injury to the patient. The recognition of CPR-related trauma forms an important part of postresuscitation care. Rib fractures, skin burns and abrasions, and upper airway trauma are relatively common injuries during CPR. Less-common injuries include trauma to the liver and spleen, vertebral fractures and intrathoracic haemorrhage.

Even when CPR is performed correctly, certain injuries may occur. For this reason, the patient must always be assessed for CPR-related trauma following a successful resuscitation. In addition to a thorough physical examination, a chest X-ray should be performed to look for evidence of bony injury, aspiration of gastric contents, pneumothorax or haemothorax. The patient's temperature is monitored closely and any symptoms or signs that may develop are carefully assessed.

SURVIVAL FOLLOWING CPR

Prediction of survival following CPR is fraught with difficulty. The outcome depends upon many different factors, such as patient characteristics, type of arrest, place of arrest and the time taken before commencing CPR. In addition, many patients who survive the initial attempt will nonetheless die before leaving hospital.

In the BRESUS study (Tunstall-Pedoe *et al.*, 1992), which reviewed the outcomes of 3765 resuscitation attempts in British hospitals, for every 16 patients on whom CPR was attempted, six survived the initial attempt, four were alive 24 h later, three left hospital, but only two were still alive after 1 year. At 1 year, the survival of patients whose initial arrest occurred outside hospital was less than half that of patients who arrested in hospital.

Patients who survive a cardiopulmonary arrest may be left with disabilities secondary to neurological impairment, and so quality of life must be taken into account as well as overall survival.

WITHHOLDING AND STOPPING CPR

The delivery of effective CPR has been made easier by the development of treatment protocols based upon reviews of current evidence. However, there are many issues that often need to be addressed but which are more difficult to reduce to a simple algorithm. These include when not to commence CPR or, having begun, when to stop. Despite the complex clinical, moral and legal considerations involved,

BOX 19.6 CRITERIA FOR WITHHOLDING CPR

- CPR refused by a patient capable of informed consent
- CPR judged to be against best interests of a patient unable to give informed consent
- CPR almost certain to prove futile

attempts have been made to formulate guidelines that will help clinicians through this often difficult area.

One set of guideline proposals, put forward by Doyal and Wilsher (1993), suggests three occasions when withholding CPR may be considered acceptable (Box 19.6). First, CPR may be withheld if patients who are judged competent to give informed consent refuse resuscitation. Second, if a patient is not competent to give consent and CPR is regarded as being against the patient's best interests (e.g. if the patient is likely to die soon from an irreversible cause), resuscitation may be withheld. Third, CPR may be withheld if it is almost certain to prove futile. However, there has to be a good deal of supporting evidence to justify withholding CPR for this reason.

Following these recommendations would involve, on many occasions, discussing CPR with patients in advance. Such discussions, which are relatively common in the USA, should be conducted sensitively but, at the same time, patients (and relatives) should be given a realistic view of the likely outcome. British and American doctors and nursing staff tend to have overoptimistic expectations of survival from CPR (Wagg *et al.*, 1995).

Decisions to withhold CPR should be made by senior members of the medical team after discussion with medical and nursing colleagues. The decision must be clearly documented in the medical and nursing notes, together with the time, date and reason for the decision. The decision should be reviewed every 24 h.

Once CPR has been commenced, how long should the attempt continue? This question cannot be answered with rigid recommendations as circumstances vary from case to case, but some useful general guidelines can be given.

CPR should not normally be abandoned while a patient remains in VF, unless the attempt was inappropriate to begin with. In addition, under certain circumstances (e.g. hypothermia, near-drowning or drug overdose), it may be justified to continue CPR for over an hour.

Conversely, it is rare for a patient to be successfully resuscitated following 15 min of asystole. Recovery is also infrequent when an arrest is unwitnessed or of unknown duration before CPR was commenced. Those who arrest in the community, and have received adequate attempts at resuscitation before reaching hospital, are also unlikely to recover with further resuscitation attempts in the hospital. Assessing a patient's pupillary reflexes is of no value in deciding whether or not to continue CPR.

TRAINING IN CPR

Despite the gradual refinement of CPR guidelines over recent years, it remains a procedure that is frequently unsuccessful. To increase the number of lives saved, ways need to be found to improve the effectiveness of CPR and to extend its availability.

Sufficient training should be given to all medical, nursing and paramedical staff to ensure that they possess the skills needed to deliver effective CPR. The survival of patients following a cardiopulmonary arrest correlates with the skills of the team performing CPR. However, training personnel just once is not adequate. Skills wane and guidelines change with the passage of time. 'Refresher' courses should therefore be provided at 6-monthly intervals (Berden *et al.*, 1993).

Lives can also be saved by making advanced life support available in the community, as it is estimated that every minute of delay in defibrillation reduces a patient's chances of survival by 5%. Many ambulance crews are therefore now trained in advanced as well as basic life support and carry the necessary drugs and equipment to deliver advanced life support outside the hospital.

To extend the availability of CPR, training in basic life support should not be restricted to health care personnel. Survival from cardiopulmonary arrest is greater when a bystander starts resuscitation. It is estimated that a community CPR training programme would, realistically, save up to six lives per 100 000 of the adult population per year (Weston *et al.*, 1994).

REFERENCES

Advanced Life Support Working Party of the European Resuscitation Council. 1992: Guidelines for advanced life support. *Resuscitation* **24**, 111–21.

Basic Life Support Working Group of the European Resuscitation Council. 1993: Guidelines for basic life support. *British Medical Journal* **306**, 1587–9.

Basic Life Support Working Party of the European Resuscitation Council. 1992: Guidelines for basic life support. *Resuscitation* **24**, 103–10.

Berden, H.J., Willems, F.F., Hendrick, J.M.A., Pijls, N.H.J. and Knape, J.T.A. 1993: How frequently should basic cardiopulmonary resuscitation training be repeated to maintain adequate skills? *British Medical Journal* **306**, 1576–7.

David, J. and Prior-Willeard, P.F.S. 1993: Resuscitation skills of MRCP candidates. *British Medical Journal* **306**, 1578–9.

Doyal, L. and Wilsher, D. 1993: Withholding cardiopulmonary resuscitation: proposals for formal guidelines. *British Medical Journal* **306**, 1593–6.

Safar, P. 1984: Recent advances in cardiopulmonary–cerebral resuscitation: a review. *Annals of Emergency Medicine* **13**, 856–62.

Tunstall-Pedoe, H., Bailey, L., Chamberlain, D.A., Marsden, A.K., Ward, M.E. and Zideman, D.A. 1992: Survey of 3765 cardiopulmonary resuscitations in British hospitals (the BRESUS study): methods and overall results. *British Medical Journal* **304**, 1347–51.

Wagg, A., Kinirons, M. and Stewart, K. 1995: Cardiopulmonary resuscitation: doctors and nurses expect too much. *Journal of the Royal College of Physicians of London* **29**, 20–4.

Weston, C.F.M., Hughes, D.W. and Donnelly, M.D.I. 1994: Potential impact upon community mortality rates of training citizens in cardiopulmonary resuscitation. *Journal of the Royal College of Physicians of London* **28**, 402–6.

20

Heimlich Manoeuvre

INTRODUCTION

Choking claimed the lives of 331 people in England and Wales in 1992, 17 of whom were children (OPCS, 1993). Anything that can enter and obstruct the airway can cause choking. In adults, the offending item is most commonly a piece of food; children, on the other hand, are not very particular about what they place in their mouths and can choke on a variety of small household objects.

As with all medical emergencies, choking requires prompt action in order to save lives. It is therefore important to recognize immediately the signs that accompany choking (Box 20.1).

The choking casualty may grip their throat. With complete obstruction of the airway, they will not be able to breathe or to speak, and so one of the most striking features is their complete silence. The skin may become cyanosed, particularly around the lips, and the person may make exaggerated efforts to take a breath. Eventually, the casualty will lose consciousness.

A number of techniques are available that allow others to assist a choking casualty to clear the obstruction from their airway. However, the role of each technique (and the order in which they should be used) remains controversial, and recommendations vary from country to country. In the UK, for example, first aiders are taught to perform both back blows and the Heimlich manoeuvre (Marsden et al.,

BOX 20.1 SIGNS THAT MAY ACCOMPANY CHOKING

- Casualty grips throat
- Complete silence
- Cyanosis
- Exaggerated efforts to breathe
- Unconsciousness

1992). In contrast, the American Heart Association recommends that, for the sake of simplicity, only the Heimlich manoeuvre is taught to the general public (Caroline, 1995).

There are advantages in minimizing the number of alternative first aid procedures taught to the lay public. However, health care professionals should be proficient in a number of different methods in order to be able to adapt their techniques according to the circumstances. This chapter will therefore describe not only the Heimlich manoeuvre but also a number of alternative methods for treating choking. The most appropriate treatment strategy will depend upon whether the casualty is initially conscious or unconscious.

THE CONSCIOUS CASUALTY

If the casualty is conscious they may be able to cough and, if so, this should be encouraged. In attempting to cough, the casualty is using the respiratory muscles to generate maximum pressure within the lungs in an attempt to expel the obstruction from their airway.

Should coughing fail to clear the airway, lean the casualty forwards (over a chair if available) so that the head is below the level of the chest. Deliver a series of up to five back blows firmly with the heel of the hand between the shoulder blades, as illustrated in Fig. 20.1.

If this fails, perform abdominal thrusts (the Heimlich manoeuvre). If the casualty is still conscious, ask them to stand or sit while you stand or kneel behind them. One arm is placed around the casualty's upper abdomen and a fist is made with the hand, so that the thumb is lying against the casualty's abdomen, halfway between the navel and xiphisternum.

Then, the other arm is brought around the other side of the casualty and the fist is held with the other

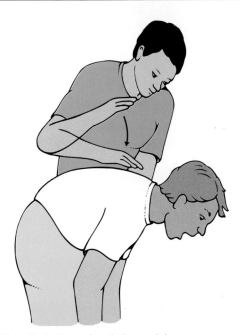

FIG 20.1   Back blows for choking adults.

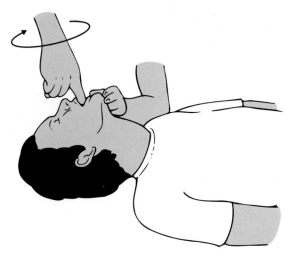

FIG 20.3   Finger sweep.

hand. Next, pull both hands towards yourself so that a firm thrust, upwards and inwards, is delivered into the casualty's upper abdomen (Fig. 20.2). This manoeuvre should also be performed up to five times in succession.

If the casualty's airway remains obstructed despite abdominal thrusts, perform a further series of five back blows. The cycle of abdominal thrusts and back blows is continued until the obstruction is expelled or until the casualty loses consciousness.

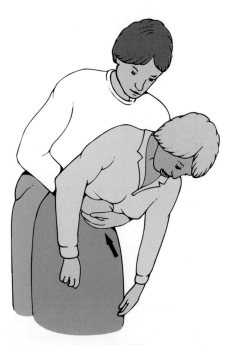

FIG 20.2   Abdominal thrust (Heimlich manoeuvre).

THE UNCONSCIOUS CASUALTY

If the casualty loses consciousness at any point, position them on their back with the mouth open, and carry out a finger sweep (Fig. 20.3). To do this, the index finger is inserted into the casualty's mouth, sweeping it around towards the back of the tongue, to see if the obstruction can be hooked out. It cannot be overemphasized that finger sweeps must be performed in a careful manner – overzealous poking around can lead to trauma and push the obstruction further down the airway.

If a finger sweep fails to dislodge the obstruction, the casualty's head is tilted backwards and the chin lifted to commence expired air respiration, as described in Chapter 19.

If the airway is still completely obstructed, expired air respiration will prove to be impossible. Roll the casualty towards you so that the person is lying on their side against your leg. Five back blows are administered (Fig. 20.4) and, again, a finger sweep is performed to see if the obstruction has been dislodged. If not, the casualty is rolled back again so that the person is lying supine, and a further series of abdominal thrusts performed.

To perform abdominal thrusts on a casualty lying supine, one can position oneself either kneeling alongside or straddling the casualty. Whichever position one adopts, the heel of one hand is placed midway between the casualty's navel and xiphisternum and the other hand is placed on top. Both hands are used to thrust firmly, inwards and upwards, and the manoeuvre is repeated up to five times (Fig. 20.5).

Once again, a finger sweep is performed. Expired air respiration is reattempted and, if this again fails, the cycle of back blows, abdominal thrusts and

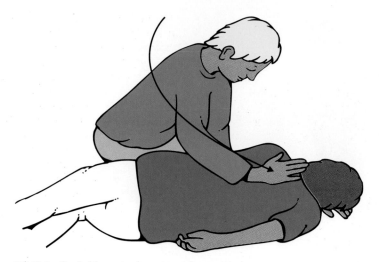

FIG 20.4   Back blows in the unconscious patient.

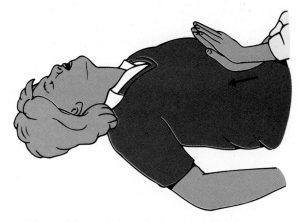

FIG 20.5   Abdominal thrust in the unconscious patient.

expired air respiration is repeated continuously. *Remember to carry out a finger sweep* after each series of back blows and abdominal thrusts to check whether the obstruction has been dislodged.

Sometimes, a choking casualty will already have become unconscious by the time assistance arrives. If the choking was not witnessed and so the cause of the loss of consciousness is initially unknown, basic life support is commenced as described in Chapter 19.

If the casualty has lost consciousness because of complete obstruction of the airway, expired air respiration will prove impossible. If this is the case, first of all check that you are correctly attempting to open the airway with a head tilt and chin lift manoeuvre and then try expired air respiration again. Repeated failure to ventilate the casualty successfully, despite an adequate head tilt and chin lift, suggests the presence of an obstruction further down the airway.

If choking is suspected, a finger sweep should be performed, if not already done, and then the casualty

rolled towards the rescuer so that five back blows can be administered, followed by another finger sweep, then a series of five abdominal thrusts and a further finger sweep. The cycle of expired air respiration, back blows and abdominal thrusts with intervening finger sweeps should be repeated continuously, as described earlier.

The obstruction may be expelled and the casualty begin to breathe spontaneously at any point during the cycle. If this occurs, the casualty should be placed in the recovery position and arrangements made for their transfer to hospital.

CHOKING IN CHILDREN

Choking is a relatively common occurrence in young children because of their habit of placing small objects in the mouth. However, it must be remembered that *foreign bodies are not the only cause of airway obstruction in young children*. Epiglottitis is a potentially fatal condition that requires urgent hospital treatment; in this condition, mistaken attempts to look for or remove foreign bodies can have disastrous consequences. For this reason, it is just as important in children as in adults to assess the situation carefully in order to reach a diagnosis.

Even when airway obstruction is caused by a foreign body, its removal has to be performed with great care in children. Finger sweeps are extremely hazardous, and can lead to trauma and displacement of the object further down the airway. Therefore, *finger sweeps must not be performed in children and infants*. No attempt should be made to remove an object unless it can clearly be seen in the child's mouth and can be easily and safely removed.

As with adults, the child who is choking on a foreign body but is still able to cough should be

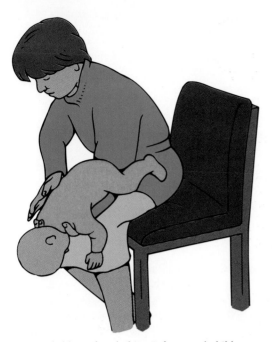

FIG 20.6   Back blows for choking infants and children.

encouraged to do so. If the child is unable to cough, or it is proving ineffective, the rescuer should kneel or sit down and invert the child over their knee (Fig. 20.6). Five back blows are then delivered in the same position as described for adults, albeit more gently.

In children over 5 years of age, the abdominal thrust may be used. The rescuer positions themself with the child either standing in front of them or sitting on their lap, facing forwards. One arm is placed around the child so that the thumb lies between the navel and xiphisternum. The other hand is used to support the child's back. Then, a thrust is delivered, inwards and upwards, but using much less pressure than one would use for an adult. The procedure may be repeated if necessary.

Unconscious children may be positioned in the same way as adults, but, again, only one hand should be used to deliver abdominal thrusts and less force should be used. Abdominal thrusts should not be used on children and infants under the age of 5 years as trauma to the abdominal organs can result.

REFERENCES

Caroline, N.L. 1995: *Emergency care in the streets*, 5th edn. Boston, MA: Little, Brown.

Marsden, A.K., Moffat, C. and Scott, R. 1992: *First aid manual – the authorised manual of St John Ambulance, St Andrew's Ambulance Association and the British Red Cross*, 6th edn. London: Dorling Kindersley.

OPCS. 1993: *Mortality statistics 1992 (cause) – England & Wales*. London: HMSO.

21

Local Anaesthesia

INTRODUCTION

Local anaesthetics may be used to provide analgesia during painful procedures (e.g. suturing of wounds, insertion of chest drains, etc.), for postoperative analgesia and for the treatment of chronic pain. Used as the sole technique for surgical procedures, the complications of general anaesthesia are avoided: the patient is able to remain conscious and respiration is not depressed. However, safe use of these techniques depends on a knowledge of anatomy, the pharmacology of the local anaesthetic agents and the ability to prevent and treat local anaesthetic toxicity. Local anaesthetics may be administered via several routes: topically (e.g. EMLA cream), by infiltration, intravenously (Bier's block), spinally or epidurally.

PRELIMINARY CONSIDERATIONS

The procedure should be explained to the patient and contraindications excluded (e.g. local anaesthetic allergy). Local anaesthetics should not be injected into inflamed or infected tissues. For major local anaesthetic procedures, trained assistance should be available and there should be facilities for resuscitation.

All equipment should be checked, together with the dose of local anaesthetic being injected (a 1% solution contains 10 mg/mL). An intravenous cannula

BOX 21.1 EFFECTS OF ADRENALINE ADDED TO LOCAL ANAESTHETIC SOLUTIONS

■ Prolongs duration of anaesthesia
■ Reduces systemic absorption
■ Increases the intensity of the block
■ Reduces surgical bleeding

should be sited if large volumes of local anaesthetic are to be injected. Aspiration should precede injection of local anaesthetic solutions to avoid intravascular injection, and verbal contact should be maintained with the patient. Intraneural injection is painful and may result in nerve damage.

Pharmacology of local anaesthetic agents

Pharmacologically, local anaesthetics are divided into two groups depending on whether the intermediate chain connecting the lipophilic head and the hydrophilic tail contains either an *ester* or an *amide*. Hypersensitivity reactions occur mainly with the ester group (Table 21.1). Local anaesthetics are usually injected as water-soluble acid solutions of the hydrochloric salt. The smaller the nerve fibre, the more sensitive it is to blockade. A differential block may occur whereby the smaller fibres carrying pain sensation and autonomic impulses are blocked, sparing coarse touch and movement.

The onset, duration and maximum dose of some local anaesthetic agents are given in Table 21.1. The onset time of conduction block depends upon the degree of ionization of the drug, its lipid solubility and the dose or concentration used. The addition of bicarbonate to local anaesthetic solutions increases the percentage of the free base and thereby increases the onset time. The duration of action of local anaesthetics is believed to be related primarily to their degree of protein binding. For example, bupivacaine, which is 97% protein bound, has a long duration of action.

Adrenaline has a number of beneficial effects when added to local anaesthetic solutions (Box 21.1). However, adrenaline should not be added to injections used in digits and appendages. The maximum dose is 500 µg and it is essential not to exceed a concentration of 1/200 000 if more than 50 mL of solution is to be injected.

TABLE 21.1   Local anaesthetic drugs: onset, duration and maximum dose

DRUG	ONSET	DURATION[a] (min)	MAXIMUM DOSE (mg/kg)
Esters			
Procaine	Slow	Short (45–60)	11–14[b]
2-Chloroprocaine[c]	Fast	Short (30–45)	15
Tetracaine	Slow	Long (60–180)	1.0–1.5
Amides			
Lignocaine	Fast	Moderate (60–120)	4–7[b]
Mepivacaine[c]	Fast	Moderate (90–120)	4–7[b]
Prilocaine	Fast	Moderate (60–120)	7–8[b]
Bupivacaine	Slow	Long (240–480)	2
Etidocaine[c]	Fast	Long (240–480)	4

[a]After infiltration.
[b]With adrenaline.
[c]Not available in the UK.

Local anaesthetic systemic toxicity

Systemic toxicity may follow either absorption of local anaesthetic from the site of injection or inadvertent intravenous injection. Factors affecting local anaesthetic toxicity are given in Box 21.2. Adrenaline may be used to reduce the rate of vascular absorption of local anaesthetic solutions. Local anaesthetic toxicity primarily involves the central nervous and cardiovascular systems; the symptoms and signs are given in Box 21.3. Bupivacaine, in particular, may produce severe cardiac arrhythmias necessitating prolonged cardiopulmonary resuscitation and the use of bretylium tosylate. Steps which should be taken to avoid systemic toxicity are given in Box 21.4. Treatment consists primarily of maintaining an adequate airway and oxygenation, and terminating seizures (Box 21.5).

BOX 21.2   FACTORS AFFECTING LOCAL ANAESTHETIC TOXICITY

▪ Dose of local anaesthetic injected
▪ Site of injection
    (absorption: intercostals > epidural > subcutaneous)
▪ Drug used
▪ Speed of injection
▪ Addition of adrenaline

BOX 21.3   SYMPTOMS AND SIGNS OF LOCAL ANAESTHETIC TOXICITY

▪ Circumoral and tongue numbness
▪ Light-headedness, tinnitus
▪ Visual disturbances
▪ Irrational behaviour and speech
▪ Muscle twitching
▪ Convulsions
▪ Unconsciousness
▪ Coma
▪ Respiratory arrest
▪ CVS depression

BOX 21.4   PREVENTION OF TOXICITY

▪ Do not exceed the recommended maximum dose
▪ Aspirate before injecting the local anaesthetic
▪ Use local anaesthetics with a low toxicity
▪ Inject the drug slowly while maintaining verbal contact with the patient

BOX 21.5   TREATMENT OF TOXICITY

Airway
▪ Maintain the airway
▪ Give 100% oxygen via a face mask

Breathing
▪ Bag and mask ventilation
▪ Tracheal intubation may be necessary

Circulation
▪ Cardiac compressions if the patient is pulseless
▪ Vasopressors may be necessary

Control convulsions
▪ Diazepam (2–5 mg IV)
▪ Thiopentone (150–200 mg IV)

TECHNIQUE

Topical anaesthesia

Local anaesthetics may be applied topically to sites including the skin, eye, tympanic membrane, gingival mucosa, tracheobronchial membrane and rectum.

EMLA cream consists of a mixture of prilocaine and lignocaine. It is used to provide analgesia during a number of procedures, such as venepuncture, venous and arterial cannulation and superficial skin surgery. The EMLA cream is applied 1 h before the procedure and covered with an occlusive dressing. Usually, 1–2 g of the cream are applied per 10 cm^2 area of skin.

Lignocaine gel is used to provide analgesia during urethral catheterization and has also been used to provide analgesia following circumcision.

Infiltration of local anaesthetic

A weal is raised by injecting the local anaesthetic solution via a small-gauge needle, and then a larger-gauge needle is used to inject the main volume of solution. Each injection is made at sites already anaesthetized. For painless skin incisions, infiltration should be intradermal as well as subcutaneous. The local anaesthetic should be injected while the needle is moving in order to reduce the risk of intravascular injection. When large areas are to be anaesthetized, large volumes of dilute solutions should be used.

Digital nerve block

The finger is supplied by two ventral and two dorsal nerves. Injections are made at the level of the metacarpal heads, using 1–2 mL of local anaesthetic on each side. Local anaesthetic solutions containing adrenaline should not be used. The procedure for the toe is the same as that for the finger.

Intercostal nerve block

Intercostal nerve blocks may be used to provide analgesia following rib fractures, herpetic neuralgia and to treat pain after thoracic or abdominal surgery.

The block may be performed by injections at the angle of the rib (with the patient in the lateral or prone positions) or at the mid-axillary line (with the patient in the supine position). The arm is raised above the head to elevate the scapula and the rib is palpated between the index and middle fingers. A 22 G needle attached to a syringe is inserted between the fingers and advanced until it contacts the rib (see Fig. 15.3, p. 79). The needle should be directed 20° cephalad. The needle is then walked down the rib until it slides under the inferior edge of the rib. It should then be advanced 2–3 mm so that the tip rests near the subcostal groove. Three to four millilitres of local anaesthetic is then injected. Pneumothorax is a possible complication although it is uncommon provided the needle is kept in close proximity to the rib.

Nerve blocks at the wrist

The terminal branches of the ulnar, median and radial nerves are all easily blocked at the wrist and this approach may be used to perform surgery on the hand.

The median nerve lies between the palmaris longus tendon and the flexor carpi radialis tendon. A 25 G needle is used to inject 2–5 mL of local anaesthetic just lateral and deep to the palmaris longus tendon.

The ulnar nerve may be similarly blocked by an injection just lateral to the flexor carpi ulnaris tendon at the level of the styloid process of the ulnar bone.

The radial nerve can be blocked by subcutaneous infiltration between the radial artery anteriorly and the extensor carpi radialis tendon posteriorly.

Femoral nerve block

A femoral nerve block is useful to provide analgesia for skin surgery of the upper thigh (e.g. skin graft harvesting) or following fracture of the femur.

The inguinal ligament runs between the anterior superior iliac ligament and the pubic tubercle. The femoral artery is palpated as it passes behind the midpoint of the ligament. A 22 G, 1/2 to 1 in needle is inserted just below the ligament, 1 cm lateral to the artery, and directed superiorly (Fig. 21.1). Once paraesthesia is obtained, 10–15 mL of local anaesthetic solution is injected. If larger volumes of solution are used (at least 20 mL) and pressure is applied below the needle, proximal spread of the solution may also block the lateral femoral cutaneous and obturator nerves. This so-called 'three-in-one block' may be used for anaesthesia of the anterior thigh and for procedures on the knee.

Intravenous regional anaesthesia (Bier's block)

This technique is popular for procedures on the upper limb (e.g. manipulation of fractures) but should only be used by experienced clinicians and preferably by an anaesthetist. The technique involves the intravenous injection of local anaesthetic into an exsanguinated limb. An intravenous cannula is placed in a

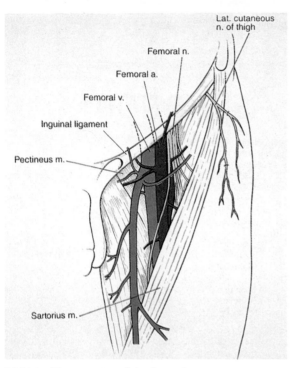

FIG 21.1 The anatomy of the femoral nerve.

vein on the dorsum of the hand of the limb to be blocked. Antecubital veins should not be used. Venous access should be established in the opposite arm. A tourniquet is applied to the upper arm and the limb is exsanguinated, either by applying an Esmarch bandage or by elevating the limb for 2 min with compression applied to the brachial artery. The cuff of the tourniquet is inflated to 100 mmHg above the systolic blood pressure and the cuff pressure should be monitored throughout the procedure. The cuff should not be deflated for at least 20 min after injection. Prilocaine is the drug of choice because of its low systemic toxicity, and 40 mL is the usual adult dose which is injected slowly.

Local anaesthetic toxicity is a serious potential problem, usually due to equipment failure or faulty technique.

FURTHER READING

Covino, B.G. 1993: Pharmacology of local anaesthetic agents. In Rogers, M.C., Tinker, J.H., Covino, B.G. and Longnecker, D.E. (eds), *Principles and practice of anesthesiology*. St Louis, MO: Mosby Year Book, 1235–7.

Gajraj, N.M. Pennant, J.H. and Watcha, M.F. 1994: Eutectic mixture of local anesthetics (EMLA) cream. *Anesthesia and Analgesia* **78**, 574–83.

Katz, J. 1994: *Atlas of regional anesthesia*. Connecticut: Appleton & Lange.

Scott, D.B. 1989: *Techniques of regional anaesthesia*. Connecticut: Appleton & Lange.

Wildsmith, J.A.W. and Armitage, E.N. 1987: *Principles and practice of regional anaesthesia*. London: Churchill Livingstone.

22

Bone Marrow Aspiration and Trephine Biopsy

INTRODUCTION

Needle aspiration and trephine biopsy of bone marrow are fundamental to the investigation of patients with haematological disease. They are also of diagnostic value in general medical and surgical fields. The techniques can be quickly and easily performed in the clinic or at the bedside. However, the quality of the diagnostic material obtained is determined by the practices employed. This chapter is intended as a guide to the procedures which should consistently provide adequate diagnostic material.

INDICATIONS

Bone marrow aspiration (BMA) and trephine biopsy are indicated for any disturbance of the peripheral blood picture that is not readily explained by other means. They allow assessment of both the quantity and quality of haematopoiesis and thus help to differentiate

between conditions inseparable by peripheral blood examination alone. Trephine biopsy is particularly useful for identifying infiltration of the bone marrow by lymphoid or non-haematological malignancy. Thus, this procedure is included in the staging process of some tumours (e.g. Hodgkin's disease or neuroblastoma). Finally, in the context of 'pyrexia of unknown origin', BMA and trephine biopsy may also prove diagnostic (e.g. marrow culture for tuberculosis and marrow morphology for leishmaniasis).

CONTRAINDICATIONS

Contraindications to BMA and trephine biopsy are few. In general, a biopsy should not be taken from a site with overlying skin sepsis (risk of osteomyelitis). Sternal body BMA is relatively contraindicated in suspected myeloma because of the possible risk of fracture if the sternum is weakened by lytic deposits.

Thrombocytopenia or anticoagulation are not contraindications. However, patients with a severe congenital coagulopathy, such as haemophilia A, should have appropriate factor replacement prior to the procedure.

TECHNIQUE

Patient explanation

Many patients have a preconception that 'bone marrow tests' are particularly painful. This is not true. The procedure can be rendered virtually pain

BOX 22.1   INDICATIONS FOR BONE MARROW ASPIRATION AND TREPHINE BIOPSY

- Unexplained anaemia
- Unexplained leucopenia or leucocytosis
- Unexplained thrombocytopenia or thrombocytosis
- Suspected marrow infiltration/staging of malignancy
- Pyrexia of unknown origin

free by the adequate use of local anaesthesia. However, there are two points during the procedure that produce transient pain which cannot be avoided without general anaesthesia. First, when a vacuum is applied to the marrow cavity by the aspirating syringe, most patients experience discomfort of variable severity. Second, during trephine biopsy it is necessary to 'wiggle' the biopsy needle in order to detach the trephine core. Again, this gives rise to transient pain. If the above is adequately explained, then most patients will tolerate the procedure very well and should not be unduly concerned about undergoing a repeat procedure at a later date.

Occasional patients are particularly anxious prior to the procedure but this can be obviated by the use of an anxiolytic agent, orally or intravenously. In children, a general anaesthetic is required.

Equipment

Box 22.2 lists the minimum equipment required to perform both a BMA and a trephine biopsy. Both the aspirate (e.g. Klima or Salah) and trephine (e.g. Jamshidi) needles should be checked prior to use to ensure that the trocars fit correctly and that they are sufficiently sharp to allow easy skin puncture (Figs 22.1 and 22.2). Usually, the needles are reused following sterilization but disposable versions exist. These have the advantage that they are always sharp but they are more expensive.

Choosing a site

When performing a diagnostic BMA, it is important that a trephine biopsy is also obtained. Occasionally, the trephine core reveals an underlying cause of a condition that may be missed by an aspirate alone (e.g. lymphoma underlying immune thrombocytopenia). In adults, this limits the choice of site to either

BOX 22.2 EQUIPMENT REQUIRED FOR BONE MARROW ASPIRATION AND TREPHINE BIOPSY

- Dressing pack with lumbar puncture towel
- Skin-cleansing solution
- Sterile gloves
- Local anaesthetic
- Syringes and needles
- Aspirate needle
- Trephine needle
- Microscopy slides
- Tubes for immunophenotyping, cytogenetics and culture samples if required
- Sticking plaster or gauze and Elastoplast

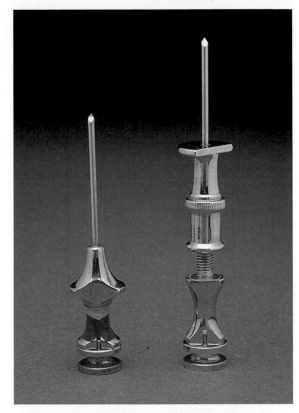

FIG 22.1 (Left) Salah and (right) Klima needles.

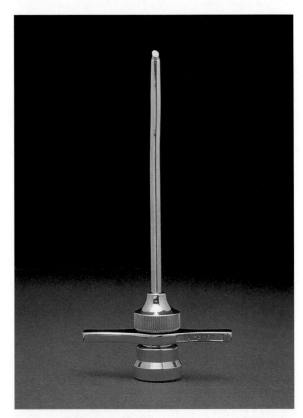

FIG 22.2 Jamshidi needle.

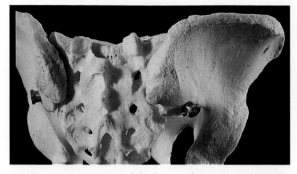

FIG 22.3 Posterior view of the bony pelvis (ignore the skeletal pins). The posterior superior iliac spine can be identified by following the iliac crest posteriorly until it is felt to widen.

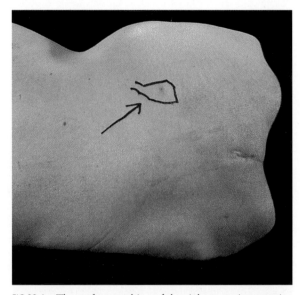

FIG 22.4 The surface marking of the right posterior superior iliac spine with the patient in the lateral position. This is often indicated by a dimple which lies about 4 cm lateral to the second spinous tubercle of the sacrum.

BOX 22.3 STEP-BY-STEP GUIDE TO BONE MARROW ASPIRATION AND TREPHINE BIOPSY

- Explain procedure to patient
- Position patient as required
- Cleanse skin
- Anaesthetize skin, subcutaneous tissue and periosteum
- Penetrate skin, subcutaneous tissue and outer cortex
- Aspirate NOT more than 0.3 mL of marrow
- Spread slides immediately for best results
- Aspirate marrow for immunophenotyping, cytogenetic analysis and culture if required
- Change to trephine needle and obtain trephine core
- Close skin

Posterior superior iliac spine aspirate and trephine biopsy

Box 22.3 gives a step-by-step account of this procedure. The PSIS should be identified by palpating the lateral aspect of the iliac crest and following it posteriorly until the crest is felt to widen. This is usually the most superficial area of bone. The surrounding skin should be cleansed with a sterilizing solution (e.g. Betadine or chlorhexidine). A lumbar puncture towel (preferably cloth) should be draped over the site. Local anaesthetic (e.g. 2% lignocaine) is then infiltrated into the skin and subcutaneous tissue. The periosteum over the PSIS should be infiltrated widely as this appears to be the most sensitive tissue. In total, anywhere between 5 and 20 mL of anaesthetic may be required.

Once anaesthetized, the aspirate needle should be applied to the skin. Steadily increasing pressure with a slight boring action allows easy penetration of the skin. Use of a scalpel blade is not required as it usually results in greater bleeding from the wound (especially in thrombocytopenic patients) and a more pronounced scar. When the periosteum is reached, a similar technique to that for skin penetration is used to breach the outer cortex of the bone. The amount of pressure required varies with the bone density and may be very little in elderly women or in those treated with corticosteroids. Cortex penetration is felt as a 'give' in the resistance to pressure. The needle should feel rigidly fixed in the bone; if not, then the needle may have slipped off the iliac spine.

Having penetrated the cortex, the trocar is withdrawn and a 10 mL syringe is attached to the needle. *Gentle* but increasing vacuum should be applied until *only the nozzle* of the syringe fills (0.3 mL). If a

the posterior superior iliac spine (PSIS) (Figs 22.3 and 22.4), the anterior superior iliac spine (ASIS) or the rarely used vertebral spinous processes. The PSIS is the favoured site unless the patient is grossly obese or unable to lie in a lateral position. If only a review marrow is required then the PSIS or the body of the sternum may be punctured. Again, the PSIS is favoured because it is a safer site in terms of needle slippage, and the patient does not have to watch the procedure.

In children up to 12 years of age, the sternum does not have an adequate marrow cavity. Hence, the PSIS is again the preferred site. In infants, the anterior aspect of the tibia may also be utilized to obtain an aspirate, but there is a risk that the tibial growth plate may be damaged.

- Ensure slides are clean – wash in spirit if necessary
- Place small drops of marrow one third of the way along slide
- Using another slide or purpose-made 'spreader', draw back onto the drop and allow it to spread laterally until two thirds of the slide width is covered
- Push 'spreader' forwards briskly at 30° to base slide

The finished product should resemble that shown in Fig. 22.5. In most instances, six slides suffice, but if the patient may be suffering from acute leukaemia, then at least 12 slides should be made. This allows diagnostic material to be sent to central trials laboratories.

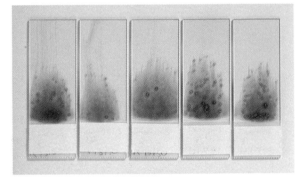

FIG 22.5   Spread marrow slides.

greater volume is extracted, the sample becomes increasingly haemodiluted, thus making subsequent interpretation more difficult. The syringe is then detached and the marrow immediately spread onto microscopy slides (Box 22.4). After spreading the films, a further 5 mL of marrow may be aspirated: 2 mL may be placed in an anticoagulated container to allow immunophenotyping studies and 3 mL may be placed in an appropriate marrow culture medium for cytogenetic analysis. It is possible to send marrow in either EDTA or citrate anticoagulated tubes to the haematology laboratory for film spreading. However, haemodilution, sample clotting and anticoagulant-induced cellular artefacts reduce the quality of the diagnostic material.

The aspirate needle is then removed, to be replaced by the trephine needle. Again, cortical penetration is achieved by increasing pressure with a slight rotary motion. Once rigidly in place, the restraining cap is unscrewed and the trocar removed. The needle should be advanced approximately 1 cm into the bone (an index finger along the barrel of the

needle can be used as a measure). The patient should then be warned of impending discomfort as the needle must now be 'wiggled' to allow detachment of the trephine core from its base. The Jamshidi needle is tapered so that its distal end has the narrowest calibre. This should trap the trephine core within the barrel of the needle. However, application of a 10 or 20 mL syringe to the proximal end of the needle and exertion of a slight vacuum will increase the frequency with which the core is actually retrieved. Once the needle is removed, the core can be extracted by pushing a second trocar into the distal end of the needle. The core is placed in a formaldehyde-based solution prior to transportation to the laboratory.

Usually, all that is required for skin closure is a sticking plaster. However, if the patient is thrombocytopenic or anticoagulated, then a pad of gauze secured by stretched Elastoplast (i.e. a pressure dressing) should be applied for 6–12 h. Postbiopsy discomfort is usually minimal but, if felt, it may be relieved by simple analgesics such as paracetamol.

Sternal aspirates

Sternal aspirates are obtained from the body of the sternum opposite the head of the third rib. The technique is essentially the same as for PSIS puncture but, in this case, a Klima needle or equivalent is essential as it has an adjustable guard. This should be set so that the needle tip does not penetrate the cortex by more than 0.5 cm. Sternal trephines are not recommended.

Vertebral spinous process aspirate and trephine

Puncture of a spinous process is rarely performed. The usual indication for this procedure is histological identification of a bone lesion that has been shown by radiological or isotopic imaging to affect the spine (e.g. suspected metastatic deposit – primary unknown).

Problems

Inaspirable marrow ('dry tap') is not infrequently encountered, usually in patients whose marrow is markedly hypercellular or fibrotic. In such situations, the trephine becomes the essential diagnostic material. However, it is possible to 'dab' the trephine core onto a glass slide and spread (to a limited degree) the marrow blood that is left behind. Alternatively, tiny amounts of marrow drawn into the barrel of the aspirate needle (but which did not reach the syringe) may be 'blown' onto a slide and spread.

CONCLUSIONS

Marrow aspirates and trephines are usually easily obtained with minimum discomfort. They are essential to the investigation of haematological disease and often useful to other specialities. The quality of the diagnostic material obtained is dependent upon avoiding haemodilution of the sample and upon adequate slide spreading. In hospitals where the haematology department provides a biopsy and/or a slide spreading service, it should be used. Where such a service is unavailable, the opportunity to practise slide spreading (e.g. with venous blood) should be taken prior to performing marrow aspirates.

23

Taking a Cervical Smear

INTRODUCTION

The purpose of a cervical smear is not to diagnose cancer but to demonstrate any lesion which may, over a period of years, develop into cervical squamous carcinoma. There are factors that predispose to development of cervical carcinoma and these are summarized in Box 23.1.

Effective mass cervical screening has resulted in a significant decrease in incidence of and mortality from cervical cancer.

BOX 23.1   HIGH-RISK FACTORS FOR CERVICAL CARCINOMA

- Early age at first intercourse
  — relative risk: <18 years = 2.5, >21 years = 1
- Multiple sexual partners
  — relative risk: 5+ partners = 2.8, 1 partner = 1
  — promiscuity of a male partner may be a factor
- Wart virus (HPV) infection
- Tobacco smoking
- Immunosuppression

PRELIMINARY CONSIDERATIONS

Who should be screened?

National guidelines operate in the UK and state that sexually active women should commence having cervical smears at age 20 years and continue until age 65 years (England and Wales) or age 60 years (Scotland).

All regions in the UK should have a computerized call and recall facility in operation, as recommended by national guidelines, to ensure maximum uptake of the screening programme.

Who should perform the screen?

Essentially, any health professional who has received adequate instruction and supervision is capable of performing a cervical smear. Bimanual examination should only be performed by those able to interpret the findings.

Cervical smear technique is of cardinal importance in obtaining a good sample and reducing the false negative rate, and is best learnt from an experienced teacher. Proceeding on the basis of having read a text or seen a video alone is not sanctionable.

TECHNIQUE

The sequence of events is summarized in Fig. 23.1 and the equipment required is shown in Fig. 23.2.

The room and equipment

The clinic room should be prepared prior to the woman's arrival. There should be a screened off area or cubicle where she can change in privacy. The examination couch should be positioned with its sides away from any walls to allow for hip flexion/abduction in the supine position. There should be a good light source at the foot of the couch, preferably a hands-free type. A female 'chaperone' must be in attendance, irrespective of the gender of the operator.

Further materials required are: vaginal specula (both Sims' and Cuscoe's in varying sizes should be to hand), a slide with a ground glass end, spatula, cervical brush, pencil, pen, request form (HMR 101/5 B), fixative (95% ethyl alcohol ± 3% glacial acetic acid) and disposable gloves.

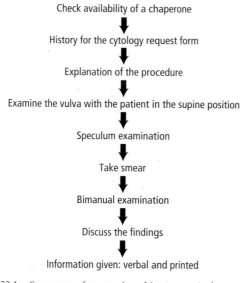

Check availability of a chaperone

↓

History for the cytology request form

↓

Explanation of the procedure

↓

Examine the vulva with the patient in the supine position

↓

Speculum examination

↓

Take smear

↓

Bimanual examination

↓

Discuss the findings

↓

Information given: verbal and printed

FIG 23.1   Sequence of events in taking a cervical smear.

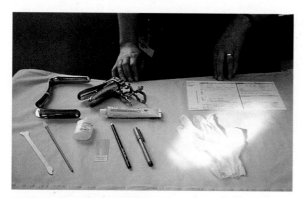

FIG 23.2   Equipment required in order to take a cervical smear. Note, a strong light is also needed. A chaperone must always be present.

History and explanation

With the clinic room prepared, it is now possible to invite the woman to enter, take a history and explain the procedure in a relaxed, unhurried atmosphere. Information needs to be gained and passed on to the cytologist and the first few minutes can be spent obtaining this and noting it on the request form (Fig. 23.3) in the appropriate boxes. Box 20 on this form should be used to record details of previous abnormal smears, previous surgery to the cervix with histological diagnoses, presence of vaginal infection and specifics of hormonal use.

This done, the procedure should be adequately explained and the woman reassured that it is quick and painless. Emphasis must be placed on the fact that this is not a test for cancer but a test to ensure that the cervix is healthy with no areas that may go on to develop cancer many years in the future. More time

will need to be spent explaining the technique to a woman attending for her first smear compared with a woman attending for, say, her seventh. A woman who is menstruating should not have a smear on that day but should reattend in 1 or 2 weeks' time. A pregnant woman may wish to defer her smear test until her postnatal follow-up and, provided she is at low risk and unlikely to default postnatally, this is reasonable. Cervical cytology is difficult to interpret in pregnancy because of activity of the transformation zone.

The woman should be shown to the changing area and asked to remove all garments below the waist.

Before proceeding to examination and smear, the slide is labelled in pencil on the ground glass with the woman's name, unit number and date of birth.

Positioning the woman and examination of the vulva

The supine position with knees drawn up and separated allows for inspection of clitoris, urethral meatus, vulval, labial and perineal skin (Fig. 23.4).

Speculum examination

This should precede digital examination to prevent contamination by lubricant and dislodgement of abnormal cells. Cuscoe's bivalve speculum is most commonly used (Fig. 23.5). If a prolapse is suspected, then Sims' speculum is used with the patient in Sims' (semi-prone) position (Fig. 23.6). In either case, the instrument is lubricated with tap water or a small amount of water-soluble gel and inserted in the direction of the vagina by aiming the tip towards L5. A Sims' speculum is used to gently retract the posterior wall of the vagina, air enters and the anterior wall and cervix are thus exposed. A Cuscoe's speculum is inserted fully, after which the blades are opened gently to expose the cervix. If there is difficulty in visualizing the cervix, then a larger Cuscoe's may be required or, if the cervix is very posterior, an easier view may be obtained by asking the woman to lift her bottom slightly off the examining couch.

Care must be taken not to traumatize the clitoris with the hinge mechanism on the Cuscoe's and to this end some recommend inserting the speculum 'upside down'.

The cervix is then inspected. Common, harmless findings include cervical ectropion (more correctly called eversion), a physiological extension of the red velvety columnar epithelium of the endocervix onto the ectocervix (often seen in pregnant women and those on the combined pill), and Nabothian cysts – mucin-filled retention cysts. Small cervical polyps may be removed after the smear has been taken and sent for histology. Cervical warts are a more sinister finding and will require referral for colposcopy and

WRITE CLEARLY WITH BALLPOINT PEN ON A **HARD SURFACE** OR BACK COPY WILL BE ILLEGIBLE

ENTER DETAILS IN BOXES OR RING APPROPRIATE NUMBERS

Fold for B

Fold for A

FORM HMR 101/5 (1989) Multi-copy

| 01 **Woman's hospital registration number** | | 02 Laboratory | 11 **Code number of laboratory** | 12 **Slide serial number** |

Fold

03 **Woman's surname** _____ Previous surname _____

First names _____

Full postal address _____ post code _____

04 **Date of birth** ___ / ___ / ___   05 **NHS number** _____

06 **A**
If hospital state consultant, clinic or ward, and hospital _____

Name and address of sender if not GP _____ post code _____

07 **B**
Name and address of GP _____ post code _____

08 **GP's FPC code**

09	GP	1	NHS hospital	4	10	1
Source of smear	NHS community clinic	2	Private	5	**LOCAL**	2
	GUM clinic	3	Other	6	**CODES**	3
				4		
				5		
				6		

Request/report for cervical or vaginal cytology – LAB. COPY

CLINICAL REPORT

17 **Reason for smear**
routine call — 1
routine recall — 2
clinically indicated — 3
previous abnormal smear — 4

18 **Specimen type**
cervical scrape — 1
other (specify) — 2

Date of:
13 this test ___ / ___ / ___
14 LMP (1st day) ___ / ___ / ___
15 last test ___ / ___ / ___
16 If no previous test please put X [ ]

19 **Condition**
pregnant — 1
post-natal (under 12 weeks) — 2
I.U.C.D. fitted — 3
taking hormones (specify in 20) — 4

20 **Clinical data** (including signs and symptoms, previous abnormal cytology with slide number, previous diagnosis and treatment)

signature

21 **CYTOLOGY REPORT**

22 **Cytological pattern**
inadequate specimen — 1
negative — 2
borderline changes — 8
mild dyskaryosis — 3
moderate dyskaryosis — 7
severe dyskaryosis — 4
severe dyskaryosis/ ? invasive carcinoma — 5
? glandular neoplasia — 6

23 **Specific infection**
trichomonas — 1
candida — 2
wart virus — 8
herpes — 3
actinomyces — 7
other (specify) — 4

24 **Management suggested**
normal recall — 1
repeat smear — 2
in ___ months
or after treatment — 3
gynaecological referral — 4
cancel recall — 5

Signature _____ date _____

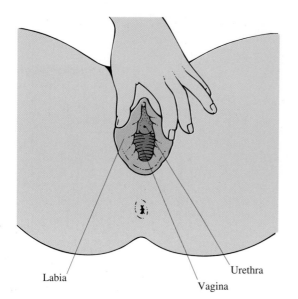

Labia

Urethra

Vagina

FIG 23.4 Positioning the woman for a cervical smear. The supine position, with flexion/abduction of the hips and flexion of the knees, allows for systematic examination of the vulva.

Cuscoe's speculum

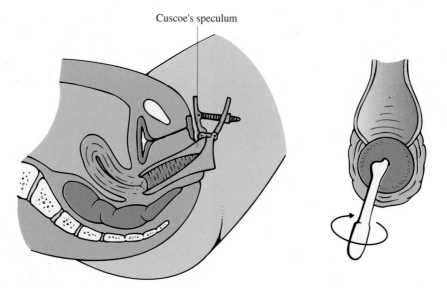

FIG 23.5 (Left) insertion of a Cuscoe's speculum and (right) collection of a cervical smear.

Sims' speculum

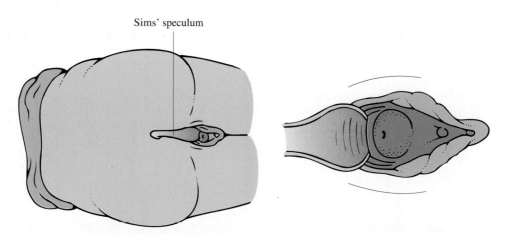

FIG 23.6 Examination in the left lateral semi-prone position with Sims' speculum inserted. This is the preferred method in cases of prolapse.

ablation. The vaginal walls, vulva, anal region and perineal skin should be examined for other warts. If warts are found, she and her partner should have STD screening and contact tracing by the GU Medicine Department. Discharges are a common finding and should be swabbed for culture.

Taking the smear

The Ayres spatula is less-and-less commonly used as a multitude of other spatulae, such as the Aylesbury spatula, have been introduced with modifications successfully aimed at increasing the efficacy of sampling. This is achieved by protruding further into the endocervical canal than the Ayres can. Some of the commoner spatulae are shown in Fig. 23.7.

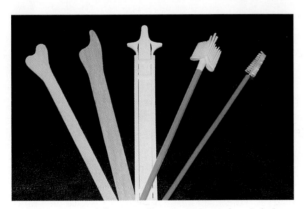

FIG 23.7 From left to right: Ayres spatula, Aylesbury spatula, Multispatula, Cervex brush and the Cytobrush.

The area that has to be sampled for the smear to be adequate is the transformation zone and squamo-columnar junction (SCJ). It is this area where neoplastic change is most likely to occur. The SCJ lies at the inner border of the transformation zone – an area where physiological change from columnar to squamous epithelium has occurred.

The spatula is inserted into the os and gently held in application to the cervix. It is then turned through 360°. If the SCJ is not visible (e.g. in a patient who has had cone biopsy), then the Cytobrush (Fig. 23.7) should be used as well. The brush end is advanced gently into the os and turned through at least one complete circle. The sample is now applied to the labelled slide as a thin layer, using longitudinal strokes rather than a circular motion, and immediately fixed.

The speculum is now removed gently with the operator inspecting the vaginal walls as they are revealed by the retreating blades.

Bimanual examination

Once the speculum is removed, two gloved fingers are inserted into the vagina and the other hand placed abdominally to push the pelvic organs onto the vaginal fingers – never the other way round. The cervix is palpated and the size, shape, consistency and position of the uterus noted. The adnexae are then palpated for evidence of any mass, and lastly the Pouch of Douglas is inspected for nodules.

At the end of the examination, the lower half of the body should be covered with a sheet and the woman asked to dress and meet back in the consultation area. She should be given a sanitary towel as sometimes spotting occurs after a smear (she should be warned of this).

The findings are discussed and the woman given the opportunity to ask questions. She should be told to allow 6 weeks for the result to reach her GP and then to telephone the surgery for the result. A normal result will be reported as 'negative'. A positive result means that abnormal changes have been found and the screening laboratory may recommend a further smear or colposcopy. It is most unlikely to be an indication of cancer. The most common reason for having to recall a woman for a repeat smear is that the initial smear was inadequate.

WHAT TO DO WITH AN ABNORMAL SMEAR

The woman should be referred for colposcopy the first time she has a moderately or severely dyskaryotic smear. A smear showing mild dyskaryotic change should be repeated after 6 months and, if still abnormal, the woman should be referred for colposcopy. There should be at least two consecutive negative smears, done 6 months apart, following a mild dyskaryotic smear result, before returning to the 3-yearly programme.

Following treatment for CIN, the first smear should be undertaken at 6 months and, if normal, repeated at 12 months. If annual smears remain normal for the next 5 years, then the woman may return to the 3-yearly screening programme.

If the woman has had a hysterectomy and has a past or current history of CIN III, then vault smears should be taken 6 months and 12 months after surgery. If these smears are normal, then further cervical screening is not required. If, however, a premalignant condition was not completely removed, then 3-yearly screening should continue after adequate treatment to the vault.

The management of women with Human Papilloma Virus (HPV) must be according to the grade of CIN present and not simply the presence of HPV.

PATIENT INFORMATION

To minimize the anxiety surrounding cervical cytology, all women undergoing screening should be provided with detailed information (verbal and printed) at all stages of screening, both before and after the smear. It is emphasized that by having regular cervical screening, signs of infection, inflammation or abnormal cell changes can be detected early and treated painlessly, thus preventing the development of more serious problems such as cancer.

Computerized call and recall of women is integral to the cervical cytology programme. Women who receive no recall may safely assume that their smear was normal. They may, if they wish, ring their doctor's surgery to confirm this, but should allow 6 weeks for the practice to receive the result.

A positive result means that abnormal changes have been seen by the screening laboratory and will require either a further smear test or colposcopy. To minimize the anxiety for those undergoing colposcopy, detailed information should be provided when first being referred, and before, during and after the procedure itself.

POSITIVE HEALTH ADVICE

This should be included in the verbal and printed information that the woman receives at the time of her smear (Fig. 23.8).

Smear tests are essential once a woman becomes sexually active. If this is done and all is well, she should have a repeat test every 3 years.

If abnormal cells are found, early treatment and regular follow-up smears are essential to ensure that a more serious condition does not develop.

The use of barrier contraception as, or as well as, the woman's regular contraceptive measures can help to protect the cervix.

Genital warts are infectious and have been linked with abnormal smears. If found, they must be treated. Cigarette smoking increases the risk of cancer of the cervix.

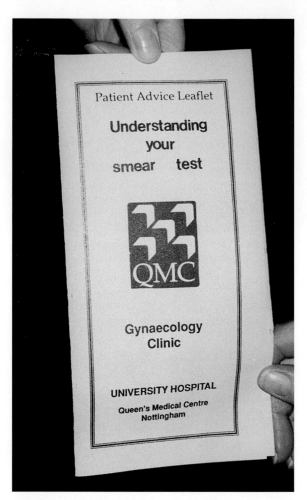

FIG 23.8 Printed information should be offered as well as verbal.

FURTHER READING

Duncan, I. D. 1992: *NHS Cervical Screening Programme. Guidelines for clinical practice and programme management.* Published by: Dr M. Gray, Oxford: National Coordinating Network.

Symonds, E.M. 1987: History and examination in gynaecology. In Symonds, E.M. (ed.) *Essential obstetrics & gynaecology.* London: Churchill Livingstone, pp. 15–20.

24

Management of Epistaxis

INTRODUCTION

Epistaxis is a common condition with an estimated prevalence of 10–13% in the general population. Although epistaxis can be a serious and even life-threatening condition, the majority of cases can be managed by patients themselves or by a GP. The more worrying cases which reach hospital tend to be the elderly. This chapter concentrates on the management of epistaxis in adults, but the general principles apply equally to children.

Anatomy

The effective management of epistaxis is dependent upon knowledge of the anatomy of the nose (Fig. 24.1). The very rich blood supply from the branches of both the internal and external carotid arteries helps in the physiological role of the nose in warming and humidifying the inspired air. Most patients with epistaxes have bleeding from the anterior nasal septum – from Kiesselbach's plexus in Little's area.

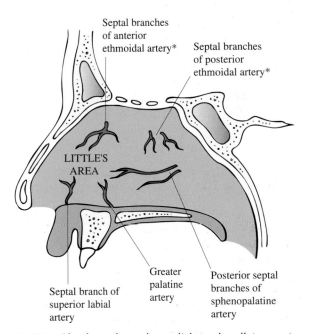

FIG 24.1   Blood supply to the medial nasal wall (septum). *From the internal carotid artery (others from the external carotid artery).

Aetiology

No obvious cause can be found for the vast majority of cases but it is important to exclude the specific factors shown in Box 24.1. Nose picking, although often vehemently denied, is a common and important cause. Patients with a coagulopathy, whether hereditary (such as haemophilia) or iatrogenic (due to warfarin treatment), must be identified early and treated accordingly. This treatment must run concurrently with the local measures to stop the bleeding, which will be described later. Although hypertension is not a cause *per se*, it does appear to increase the severity of the bleeds. It should be remembered that the anxiety generated by a severe nosebleed may elevate the blood pressure of a normotensive patient or further increase the blood pressure of a known or previously undiagnosed hypertensive. Hereditary haemorrhagic telangiectasia is an important cause of torrential epistaxes; one should look for the diagnostic lesions around the lips and tongue. The range of treatment options for this disease, both operative and non-operative, implies that none is particularly effective: examples include oestrogen therapy, laser surgery and septodermoplasty.

BOX 24.1 CAUSES OF EPISTAXIS

Systemic

Causes	*Examples*
▪ Platelet disorders	▪ Thrombocytopenia ▪ Thrombocytopathy (e.g. aspirin therapy)
▪ Vascular disorders	▪ Hereditary haemorrhagic telangiectasia
▪ Coagulation defects	▪ Haemophilia ▪ Liver disease ▪ Anticoagulant therapy
▪ Excessive thrombolysis	▪ Thrombolytic therapy ▪ Disseminated neoplasms

Local

Causes	*Examples*
▪ Idiopathic	
▪ Trauma	▪ Nose picking ▪ Direct injury ▪ Postoperative
▪ Infection	▪ Acute and chronic rhinosinusitis
▪ Neoplasia	▪ Benign: haemangioma or papilloma ▪ Malignant: carcinoma or melanoma
▪ Drugs	▪ Cocaine abuse ▪ Snuff

MANAGEMENT OF NOSEBLEEDS

Local measures for mild epistaxes

Compression over the alae nasi or soft cartilaginous portion of the nose (with the patient sitting up and leaning forwards to prevent blood from running back into the pharynx) for 10 to 15 min will stop most nosebleeds. Ice-packs across the nose and sucking ice may also help. It was found that over 50% of trained medical and nursing staff of a major teaching hospital's Accident and Emergency Department were unaware of this simple manoeuvre (McGarry and Moulton, 1993). In a study in children, there was found to be no significant difference between treatment with an antiseptic nasal cream (Naseptin) and silver nitrate cautery (Ruddy *et al.*, 1991) so the less traumatic cream application to the anterior septum is to be recommended.

Immediate measures in severe epistaxes

The severity of nosebleeds varies from trivial to life threatening. In the latter group, it is essential to adopt a systematic approach (*see* Chapter 19). First, one must ensure that the airway is secure and free from clots or foreign bodies such as dentures. Second, breathing is assessed and oxygen given if necessary. Third, one should make sure that the circulatory state is satisfactory. If the patient has bled or is bleeding significantly, intravenous colloids or crystalloids must be given whilst haemostasis is being secured. If severe bleeding continues, blood will need to be cross-matched and, where appropriate, a clotting screen performed.

Examination of the nose

The equipment needed for a proper examination of the nose is shown in Fig. 24.2. If a head mirror and light source are not available, then an auriscope with a large speculum may be used. A kidney dish should be at hand for the patient to spit into, and the doctor should be suitably protected with gloves, plastic apron and goggles if necessary. Using a Thudichum's nasal speculum to open the nasal vestibule, clots should be removed using a Frazier sucker to allow visualization of any obvious bleeding point. The oropharynx should also be examined and any clots removed using Tilley's dressing forceps.

The next step is to anaesthetize the nose and to simultaneously induce vasoconstriction using 2 mL of a solution of 10% cocaine in 1/10 000 adrenaline soaked onto cotton wool shaped into a sausage; this is then inserted into the bleeding nostril. An alternative is to use a 5–20% cocaine spray (maximum 2 mg/kg), but with active bleeding this is less effective.

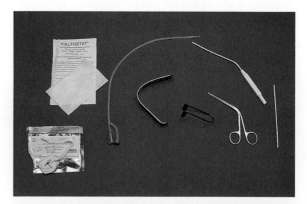

FIG 24.2   Equipment to examine the nose. From left to right: gauze impregnated with bismuth and iodoform paraffin paste, kaltostat, Foley catheter, tongue depressor, Thudichum's nasal speculum, Tilley's dressing forceps, Frazier sucker and a silver nitrate stick.

BOX 24.2 CONTROLLING EPISTAXIS

Pressure and ice in the upright position

Cautery
- Chemical (silver nitrate)
- Electrical

Packing (anterior or posterior)
- Ribbon gauze (e.g. bismuth and iodoform paraffin paste or vaseline anteriorly and gauze swab posteriorly)
- Kaltostat (calcium-sodium-alginate fibre)
- Balloons (e.g. Epistat, Foley, Brighton or Simpson)

Surgery
- Examination, cautery and packing under general anaesthesia
- Submucous resection of the nasal septum
- Arterial ligation
- Embolization

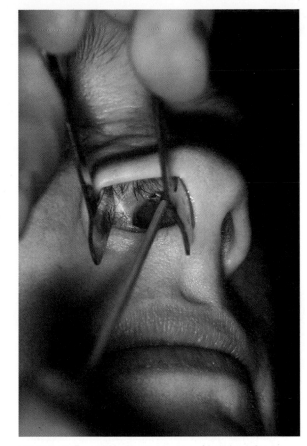

FIG 24.3 Silver nitrate cautery to nasal septum.

Haemostasis

The methods which are used are listed in Box 24.2.

Cautery

This may be chemical or electrical, the former being more suitable for use in the Accident and Emergency Department. Silver nitrate on an orange stick is commonly used (Fig. 24.3). By applying it gently around rather than on the bleeding point, haemostasis may be achieved, though it is frequently of benefit to apply firm pressure with some cotton wool on the end of a pair of Tilley's forceps, for a minute, to ensure that the grey residue is not lifted off by further bleeding. If this works, the patient should be observed for a period before being allowed home. With continuing and heavy bleeding, the patient should be admitted to a hospital.

Electrocautery should only be performed by an otorhinolaryngologist. When performed with a dissecting microscope, it has been shown to reduce the length of hospital stay and reduce the use of nasal packing. The hazards are burns to the skin and a greater risk of septal perforation. Cautery will lead to the formation of scabs; Naseptin cream applied three times a day for 2 weeks will soften the scabs and prevent infection.

Packing

When cautery fails, patients require nasal packing. This may be anterior alone or both anterior and posterior. A range of materials may be used (Box 24.2).

The most commonly used material is 1/2 in ribbon gauze soaked in bismuth, iodoform and paraffin paste (BIPP). The technique requires some fortitude and significant cooperation from the patient. The gauze is grasped 5 in from one end with a pair of Tilley's forceps and the tip of the forceps advanced along the floor of the nose to the nasopharynx. Both ends of the gauze should still be hanging from the nostril. The next layer of gauze is grasped 4 in from the nares and inserted on top of the first layer in a pleating design (Fig. 24.4). This is continued until the nasal cavity is full and the bleeding has been arrested. A bolster consisting of some rolled gauze is applied beneath the nose to retain the pack. It is kinder to pack only one nostril to allow breathing through the other side. Unfortunately, sometimes it is only possible to exert sufficient pressure on the bleeding point with bilateral packs. The pack is retained for 24 h. Some sedation (e.g. 2 mg of diazepam orally) may be required during this period. Antibiotics are not necessary, except in patients with damaged or prosthetic heart valves. Kaltostat (calcium-sodium-alginate fibre) has been found to be as effective as BIPP and is considerably easier to insert as it does not involve layering.

Intranasal balloon catheters may be used to control haemorrhage. Several types are available

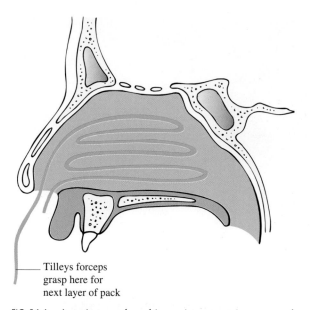

Tilleys forceps
grasp here for
next layer of pack

FIG 24.4 Anterior nasal packing using gauze impregnated with BIPP. Note pleating of gauze.

including the Epistat nasal catheter, the Simpson plug and the Brighton balloon. They all work by a combination of tamponade, choanal occlusion, direct pressure on bleeding points and pressure on the turbinate arteries.

Additional posterior packing may be necessary when there is heavy blood loss into the nasopharynx. The simplest way to achieve this is with a Foley catheter. This is inserted into the nasopharynx via the anterior nares. The position should be checked by advancing the tip of the catheter until it is just visible in the oropharynx and then retracting it slightly. The balloon of the catheter is inflated with 5–10 mL of water and the catheter is then firmly pulled back to occlude the choana. An anterior pack is then inserted whilst an assistant keeps traction on the Foley catheter, which may finally be secured by an umbilical cord clamp with some intervening gauze to protect the skin of the nares. Packing should be avoided in cases of trauma until one can be sure that there are no nasal fractures, otherwise unstable fractures may be displaced. Most traumatic nosebleeds will stop spontaneously, but surgical reduction of the fracture may be necessary to free a trapped or bleeding vessel. One should be wary of traumatic nosebleeds which restart after a period of quiescence.

Surgery (see also Box 24.2)

Failure to control bleeding with the measures described will necessitate examination and packing under anaesthesia, and this will require experienced help. Whilst the vast majority of epistaxes can be managed without operative intervention, a small minority may need arterial ligation or embolization.

REFERENCES

McGarry, G.W. and Moulton, C. 1993: The first aid management of epistaxis by accident and emergency staff. *Archives of Emergency Medicine* 10, 298–300.

Ruddy, J., Proops, D.W., Pearman, K. and Ruddy, H. 1991: Management of epistaxis in children. *International Journal of Paediatric Otorhinolaryngology* 21, 139–42.

25

Lumbar Puncture

INTRODUCTION

Lumbar puncture is the insertion of a needle into the subarachnoid space at the lumbar level for diagnostic, therapeutic or anaesthetic purposes. This chapter focuses on diagnostic lumbar puncture in adults, where the procedure is used to obtain a sample of cerebrospinal fluid (CSF) for analysis. The fluid is removed through a needle inserted into the lumbar subarachnoid space, usually in the L3–4 or L4–5 interspace. This is well below the end of the spinal cord at the lower border of L1 (Fig. 25.1). The procedure is relatively safe if preceded by careful clinical evaluation of the patient; it should *NOT* be undertaken unless there are clear indications.

INDICATIONS

Lumbar puncture is often performed to obtain fluid for diagnostic purposes (Box 25.1), but it does have other applications.

BOX 25.1   DIAGNOSTIC APPLICATIONS OF LUMBAR PUNCTURE

- Suspected infection of the central nervous system
- Subarachnoid haemorrhage
- Demyelination
- Inflammation
- Malignant meningitis

Diagnostic indications

Suspected central nervous system infection

Suspected bacterial meningitis is an urgent indication for lumbar puncture. In this condition, treatment must be given as soon as possible and not delayed until after the lumbar puncture. In a patient with an unexplained fever or confusional state, examination of the CSF may be appropriate to exclude infections such as tuberculous meningitis, encephalitis or neurosyphilis, which are often insidious in their presentation. In immunocompromised patients, such as those with AIDS, infections with unusual organisms, such as *Cryptococcus, Toxoplasma* or *Listeria,* are not infrequent and the microbiological laboratory should be alerted appropriately.

Subarachnoid haemorrhage

If subarachnoid haemorrhage is suspected, then a computed tomography (CT) scan, if available, is the

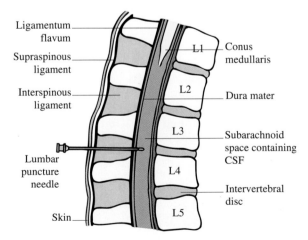

FIG 25.1   A longitudinal section through the lumbar spine. The lumbar puncture needle is inserted in the L3–4 interspace, well below the end of the spinal cord.

first line of investigation. If the scan is negative, examination of the CSF is necessary to establish the diagnosis.

Inflammation

Lumbar puncture may help to establish the diagnosis of multiple sclerosis, vasculitides and other inflammatory conditions of the central nervous system. Supportive evidence for the diagnosis of multiple sclerosis may come from examination of the CSF for lymphocytes, protein and immunoglobulins. Discrete (oligoclonal) bands are found on immunoelectrophoresis in 90% of cases but these are not specific. Oligoclonal bands are also found in sarcoidosis and syphilis.

Neoplasia

In a patient with leukaemic or carcinomatous meningitis, diagnostic cells may be found in the CSF.

Other applications of lumbar puncture

These require specialist supervision and are only mentioned briefly here.

Introduction of contrast media

The technique of lumbar puncture is used to introduce contrast medium when carrying out a myelogram.

Spinal anaesthesia

In spinal anaesthesia, lumbar puncture is performed to gain access to the subarachnoid space. An anaesthetic is then administered by this route.

Chemotherapy

A patient with leukaemia or lymphoma may need to be given drugs intrathecally. One must check, *with extreme care*, the details and dosages of any drug to be given intrathecally.

Benign intracranial hypertension (BIH)

This is the only situation where lumbar puncture maybe performed on patients with raised intracranial pressure. The diagnosis is made after other causes of raised intracranial pressure have been excluded on clinical grounds and by CT scan. The lumbar puncture is required to confirm that the CSF pressure is elevated. Treatment of BIH may involve repeated lumbar punctures with drainage of up to 30 mL of CSF on each occasion. Such measures should not be undertaken without the advice of a neurologist.

CONTRAINDICATIONS

Contraindications to lumbar puncture are listed in Box 25.2 and are described below.

BOX 25.2   CONTRAINDICATIONS TO LUMBAR PUNCTURE

■ Raised intracranial pressure
■ Spinal cord compression
■ Local sepsis
■ Bleeding disorders

Raised intracranial pressure

This is an absolute contraindication except to confirm benign intracranial hypertension. Removal of CSF may precipitate herniation of the brain downwards through the tentorial opening and the foramen magnum, leading to compression of the midbrain and medullary centres (coning).

Spinal cord compression

In this situation, lumbar puncture may lead to abrupt worsening of the cord compression.

Local sepsis

Lumbar puncture should be avoided if there is nearby infection, such as a pressure sore.

Bleeding disorders

A patient taking anticoagulants or who has a bleeding diathesis or thrombocytopenia is at risk of haemorrhage after lumbar puncture. One should undertake the procedure only if the indications are urgent and after taking measures to correct the bleeding tendency.

TECHNIQUE

A nurse's presence is essential to help position and reassure the patient, and to assist with aseptic technique.

BOX 25.3 EQUIPMENT NEEDED FOR LUMBAR PUNCTURE

- Antiseptic solution (e.g. ethanol or povidone-iodine)
- Sterile drapes and gloves
- Skin-marker pen
- 2 mL 2% lignocaine
- 2 mL syringe
- 21 G (green-hubbed) needle
- 25 G (orange-hubbed) needle
- Lumbar puncture needles
- Manometer
- Collection bottles
- Gauze squares and tape

Equipment

Before preparing the patient, it is wise to check that everything needed for the procedure is available at hand (Box 25.3). There are various types and sizes of lumbar puncture needles to choose from. The standard needles, such as the Quincke or Yale needles, have bevelled cutting edges. A 20 G or 22 G standard needle is commonly used for diagnostic lumbar puncture. These allow for free flow of CSF. The choice of needle is discussed further in connection with post lumbar puncture headache (see section on Complications).

Positioning the patient

It is worth spending some time at this stage getting the positioning right. The patient is asked to lie on the left side at the edge of a firm bed, with their knees tucked up to the chest and the spine slightly flexed (Fig. 25.2(a)). There is no need for the patient to be curled into a tight ball; this is an uncomfortable position and difficult to sustain. One pillow is placed under the head and one or two between the knees to support the top leg and upper arm. This prevents the patient from rolling forwards and ensures that the spine is straight and the back perpendicular to the surface of the bed.

An alternative position, which some clinicians prefer, is with the patient sitting upright and leaning forwards. This can be achieved by asking the patient to straddle a chair and to hold on to the back, or to sit across an examination couch with the feet on a stool, with the spine flexed and the chin on the sternum (Fig. 25.2(b)). These upright positions are particularly useful if patients have difficulty in lying flat, or are so obese that localization of the midline is difficult in the lateral position.

Once the patient is correctly positioned, the next step is to locate the fourth lumbar vertebra. A line

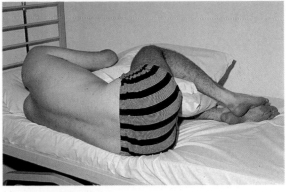

(a)

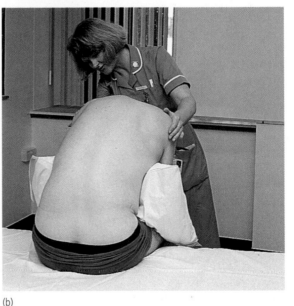

(b)

FIG 25.2   (a) The patient is positioned on their left side at the edge of the bed, with their knees drawn up and the spine slightly flexed. (b) An alternative position with the patient sitting across the examination couch with the spine flexed and the chin on the sternum.

drawn between the most cephalad parts of both iliac crests (Tuffier's line) intercepts the vertebral column at, or just below, this spine (Fig. 25.3). If only one iliac crest is used to locate L4, 30% of needles are misplaced at L2–3 or above, as opposed to only 4% when Tuffier's line is drawn (Ievins, 1991). The puncture may be made through the L3–4 or L4–5 interspace. The chosen space is identified and marked with a skin-marker pen.

Insertion of the lumbar puncture needle

At this stage, the operator washes their hands, puts on sterile gloves and lays out the equipment with the

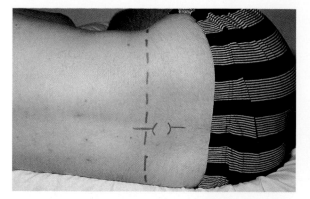

FIG 25.3   A line joining the ilic crests (Tuffier's line) intercepts the vertebral column at, or just below, the fourth
lumbar (L4) vertebral spine. The L4–5 interspace is marked.

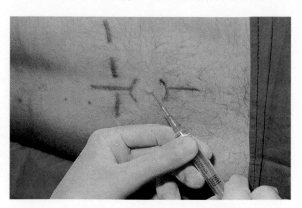

FIG 25.5   The skin is anaesthetized with 2% lignocaine
using an orange-hubbed 25 G needle.

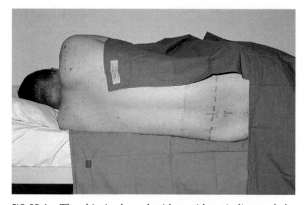

FIG 25.4   The skin is cleaned with povidone-iodine and the
patient and bed are covered with sterile drapes.

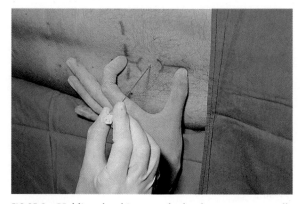

FIG 25.6   Holding the skin taut, the lumbar puncture needle
is pushed slowly but firmly through the skin.

assistance of the nurse. One should check that the
lumbar puncture needle and stylet fit together and
that the stylet does not protrude from the bevelled
cutting edge. One should also ensure that the
manometer fits onto the end of the needle. The skin
is cleaned with povidone-iodine and three drapes are
arranged (Fig. 25.4). Using an orange-hubbed 25 G
needle, a skin bleb is raised using 2% lignocaine and
then the area is infiltrated subcutaneously (Fig. 25.5).
There is no need to infiltrate the deeper tissues, which
are less pain sensitive, as this will distort the tissues
and make the procedure more difficult.

The position of the patient is checked again. Using
the index finger and thumb of the left hand (if one is
right-handed) to hold the skin taut, the lumbar
puncture needle is pushed through the skin (Fig.
25.6). If one is using a standard needle, the bevel
should be in the sagittal plane so that it separates
rather than divides the longitudinal fibres of the dura.
It is helpful to look at the needle from the side at this
point to make sure that it is perpendicular to the
patient's back. The needle is advanced gently, directing it slightly towards the patient's head, and checking that it remains at 90° to the back. If the needle

is off line, it should be withdrawn to just below the
skin and redirected. At about 4–7 cm, one will feel
the resistance of the ligamentum flavum; the needle
is advanced a little further and it will penetrate this
with a slight 'pop'. The dura mater is sometimes
breached at the same time, but one may experience a
separate resistance. The stylet is withdrawn to look
for the flow of CSF.

If no CSF emerges, the needle is rotated through
90° as a nerve root may be lying across the end. If
there is still no fluid, the stylet is replaced, the bevel
of the needle is realigned, and the needle is advanced
a millimetre or two. This process is repeated until CSF
starts to flow from the needle. If one encounters firm
resistance at any stage, the needle must not be forced
as it may be against bone or an intervertebral disc. If
the patient complains of pain down one leg, a nerve
root has probably been hit, indicating that the needle
was angled away from the midline, towards the side
of the pain. Under these circumstances, the needle
should be withdrawn completely, the position of the
patient checked and the procedure started again. One
should limit oneself to two or three attempts in one
interspace. It is wise to seek help from someone more

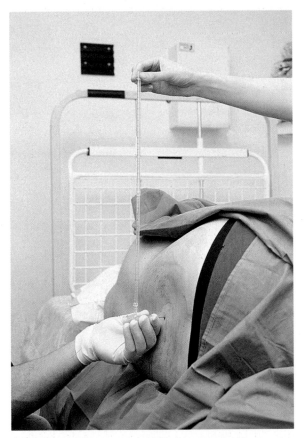

FIG 25.7 A manometer is attached to measure the opening pressure.

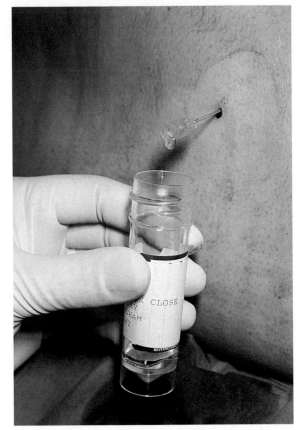

FIG 25.8 Samples of CSF are collected in sterile containers.

experienced at this stage, rather than after several spaces have been traumatized.

Manometry

When CSF appears at the end of the lumbar puncture needle, the manometer is connected. The assistant is asked to hold the top to steady it and then the reading of the opening pressure is recorded (Fig. 25.7). A normal value for the relaxed patient is between 80 and 200 mmCSF. The pressure may be higher in anxious patients but pressures of over 250 mmCSF are abnormal. In the past, jugular compression (the Queckenstedt test) has been used to test for spinal block. This test is dangerous and should no longer be used (Patten, 1996). A cough by the patient will produce a brisk 10 mm rise and fall in pressure, which is all that is needed to demonstrate the absence of spinal block.

Specimens for diagnosis

If the CSF pressure is within normal limits, the fluid is run from the manometer into a sterile container and then two further samples are collected, each of about 5 mL (Fig. 25.8). The three samples are numbered sequentially. A further sample of 2 mL is collected into a fluoride tube for measurement of CSF glucose. The CSF glucose must be interpreted in the context of the blood glucose concentration, so straight after the lumbar puncture a blood glucose level is taken to send to the laboratory with the CSF. The normal CSF glucose is 60–80% of the blood glucose.

Post lumbar puncture care

When the specimens of CSF have been collected, the needle is withdrawn and a sterile gauze dressing is applied to the puncture site. There is no need for prolonged bedrest as this does not reduce the incidence of post lumbar puncture headache (Spriggs et al., 1992). However, if headaches do occur, lying down may relieve them.

COMPLICATIONS

Lumbar puncture should be straightforward, but there are potential complications.

Failure to obtain CSF

A 'dry tap' usually results from poor positioning of the patient and consequent misdirection of the needle. One may encounter problems in directing the needle correctly in obese patients, or in those with osteoarthritic spines in whom osteophytes may impede access to the spinal canal. Neural damage and accidental puncture of an intervertebral disc, resulting in disc rupture, have occurred after misdirection of a lumbar puncture needle. A 'dry tap' is more rarely caused by blockage or malignant infiltration of the spinal canal and interruption of the flow of CSF. This can be confirmed by an MRI scan.

Abnormal CSF pressure

Careful assessment of patients before carrying out lumbar puncture will hopefully exclude most of those with abnormal CSF pressure. Occasionally, the pressure may be unexpectedly high or low. If the pressure is high, one should collect the CSF from the manometer and withdraw the needle. Intravenous access should be established in case it may be necessary to give mannitol. Expert neurological help should be sought. Help will also be needed if the pressure is very low; this may be due to spinal block or cerebellar tonsillar herniation and no attempt should be made to collect CSF, apart from that already in the manometer.

Post lumbar puncture headache

This headache is characteristically exacerbated by an upright position and relieved by lying flat. It may be severe, frontal or occipital, and associated with neck stiffness, back pain, and nausea and vomiting. It most commonly presents within 48 h of dural puncture. Post lumbar puncture headache is thought to be due to leakage of CSF through the dural puncture site into the epidural and paravertebral spaces. This leads to low CSF pressure and gravity-dependent traction on pain-sensitive structures within the cranial cavity, producing a headache. The incidence of the headache varies widely in published reports, from 2% up to 75% (Leibold *et al.*, 1993). This is because of different populations, techniques and varying criteria in diagnosing post lumbar puncture headache.

The main risk factors for post lumbar puncture headache are shown in Box 25.4. The main modifiable risk factors relate to size, type and bevel of the lumbar puncture needle. Lower rates of headache are associated with finer needles that are thought to make a smaller hole in the dura which heals more easily. The pencil-point type of needle (e.g. Sprotte or Whitacre), which separates rather than tears the dural fibres, gives a lower incidence of post lumbar puncture headache than standard needles (e.g. Quicke or Yale) of the same gauge (Lynch *et al.*, 1991).

BOX 25.4   RISK FACTORS FOR DEVELOPING POST LUMBAR PUNCTURE HEADACHE

- Young age
- Female
- Large needle size
- Bevelled needle type compared with pencil-point needle of same gauge
- Bevel of needle cutting across dural fibres
- Multiple punctures

A pencil-point needle or very fine standard needle is indicated for spinal anaesthesia, especially in a young patient. These needles are not recommended for diagnostic use as they do not allow a free flow of CSF, with resultant difficulties in measuring the opening pressure and in obtaining sufficient fluid.

The treatment of post lumbar puncture headache includes bedrest, analgesia and adequate rehydration. If these measures do not control the headache, other means are available, such as the use of an epidural blood patch (Gormley, 1960), but these methods are beyond the scope of this chapter.

Neurological complications

Serious neurological sequelae are rare. Subdural haematoma is well recognized. Subarachnoid haemorrhage, medullary and tentorial coning, meningitis and cranial nerve palsies causing diplopia, tinnitus and bilateral deafness have also been reported.

CEREBROSPINAL FLUID APPEARANCE AND INVESTIGATIONS

The appearance of the CSF may be the first clue to the diagnosis (Fig. 25.9 and Table 25.1). Normal CSF is clear and colourless. In bacterial meningitis, the CSF is yellow and cloudy because of neutrophil pleocytosis. Excess lymphocytes, as found in viral

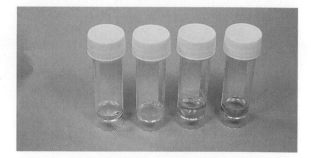

FIG 25.9   Appearances of CSF. From left to right: clear, turbid, xanthochromic and bloodstained.

TABLE 25.1 Clinical parameters of cerebrospinal fluid (CSF) in a normal individual and for a range of diseases

CONDITION	APPEARANCE	CYTOLOGY (cells/mm³)	PROTEIN (g/L)	GLUCOSE (mmol/L)
Normal	Clear and colourless	Lymphocytes <5, red cells 0	0.1–0.45	2.5–4.0 (>50% of blood glucose value)
Acute bacterial meningitis	Cloudy and yellowish or purulent	500–10 000 cells, mainly polymorphs	0.5–5.0	0–4.0
Viral meningitis	Clear or faintly turbid	5–500 cells, mainly lymphocytes	0.1–0.8	2.5–4.0
Tuberculous meningitis	Clear or opalescent	50–500 cells; mixed polymorphs and lymphocytes early, mainly lymphocytes later	0.5–1.5	0.1–4.0
Fungal meningitis	Clear or cloudy	100–1000 cells, mainly lymphocytes	0.5–1.5	0.1–4.0
Subarachnoid haemorrhage	Bloodstained Xanthochromic supernatant	>100 red cells + lymphocytic reaction	<0.5	2.5–4.0
Multiple sclerosis	Clear and colourless	<50 cells, mainly lymphocytes	0.4–0.7 (increased fraction is gamma globulin)	2.5–4.0
Malignant meningitis	Clear or faintly turbid	0–50 reactive lymphocytes ± malignant cells	0.1–5.0	0–4.0

meningitis, rarely cause visible changes. Specimens of CSF with a high protein content, for example in tuberculous meningitis, may form cobweb-like fibrin-like strands if they are allowed to stand. The CSF in spinal block is yellowish with a high protein content (Froin's syndrome).

Bloodstaining of the CSF may be due to a traumatic tap or subarachnoid haemorrhage. These can be distinguished in three ways:

1. As the CSF is collected, blood due to trauma often streams in an otherwise clear CSF. The CSF in subarachnoid haemorrhage is diffusely bloodstained.
2. A traumatic puncture is indicated by a decrease in bloodstaining (and the red cell count) in the three subsequent samples.
3. On centrifugation or standing of the CSF, the supernatant is colourless in a traumatic tap, but xanthochromic in a subarachnoid haemorrhage.

There are exceptions to this last point. The supernatant may be clear if the lumbar puncture is done within 4–6 h of the subarachnoid haemorrhage, before there has been time for the erythrocytes to lyse. In a very traumatic tap (> 100 000 red cells/μL), plasma proteins are present in sufficient concentration to cause minimum xanthochromia.

The CSF samples are sent for biochemical, bacteriological, cytological and immunological investigation as appropriate. The most frequently requested tests are listed in Box 25.5, and Table 25.1 shows the CSF findings in a number of disorders.

BOX 25.5 LABORATORY TESTS FOR THE INVESTIGATION OF SAMPLES OF CEREBROSPINAL FLUID

Microbiology
- Direct staining and microscopy
  — bacteria
  — acid-fast bacilli
  — fungi
  — protozoa
- Culture
- Serology
- Latex particle agglutination for fungi and bacterial antigens
- Polymerase chain reaction to Herpes simplex encephalitis and tuberculosis

Cytology
- Polymorph, lymphocyte and red cell counts
- Malignant cells

Chemical pathology
- Protein content
- Glucose concentration (and blood glucose concentration for comparison)

Immunology
- Immunoglobulins
- Electrophoresis for oligoclonal bands

CONCLUSIONS

Lumbar puncture should be a straightforward procedure but the indications *must be clear* and contraindications, particularly raised intracranial pressure, must be excluded. The appearances of the CSF may give a clue to the diagnosis, even before detailed laboratory analysis is available.

REFERENCES

Gormley, J.B. 1960: Treatment of post-spinal headache. *Anesthesiology* **21**, 565–6.

Ievins, F.A. 1991: Accuracy of placement of extradural needles in the L3/4 interspace: comparison of two methods of identifying L4. *British Journal of Anaesthesia* **66**, 381–2.

Leibold, R.A., Yealy, D.M., Coppola, M. and Cantees, K.K. 1993: Post-dural puncture headache: characteristics, management and prevention. *Annals of Emergency Medicine* **22**, 1863–70.

Lynch, J., Krings-Ernst, I., Strick, K., Topalidis, K., Schaaf, H. and Fiebig, M. 1991: Use of a 25 gauge Whitacre needle to reduce the incidence of post-dural puncture headache. *British Journal of Anaesthesia* **67**, 692–3.

Patten, J. 1996: *Neurological differential diagnosis*. London: Harold Starke; New York: Springer-Verlag.

Spriggs, D.A., Burn, D.J., French, J., Cartlidge, N.E.F. and Bates, D. 1992: Is bed rest useful after diagnostic lumbar puncture? *Postgraduate Medical Journal* **68**, 581–3.

Index